# THE
# EVERYTHING
## Calorie Counting Cookbook

Dear Reader,

I decided to write this book for one very simple reason: I lost 40 pounds counting calories and am continuing to count and lose. I cannot think of a better reason or a better endorsement for counting calories than this.

At first, counting calories was a great learning experience and exploration. Over time, it became tedious and then I hit the all-dreaded plateau. For six months I could not drop a single ounce, but I did some research and learned that the body gets smart, it becomes hip to your tricks, and I needed to find ways to jump-start my metabolism. I also needed to get excited about food and counting calories again in order to make it work.

This book is my journey with food. I still eat, and I eat a lot. The difference is that I now know when to stop, and I have created a book of recipes that makes it a foolproof journey each day. Enjoy!

*Paula Conway*

# Welcome to the EVERYTHING Series!

These handy, accessible books give you all you need to tackle a difficult project, gain a new hobby, comprehend a fascinating topic, prepare for an exam, or even brush up on something you learned back in school but have since forgotten.

You can read an *Everything*® book from cover to cover or just pick out the information you want from our four useful boxes: e-questions, e-facts, e-alerts, e-ssentials. We give you everything you need to know on the subject, but throw in a lot of fun stuff along the way, too.

We now have more than 400 *Everything*® books in print, spanning such wide-ranging categories as weddings, pregnancy, cooking, music instruction, foreign language, crafts, pets, New Age, and so much more. When you're done reading them all, you can finally say you know *Everything*®!

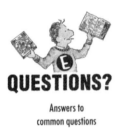

## QUESTIONS?

Answers to
common questions

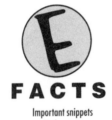

## FACTS

Important snippets
of information

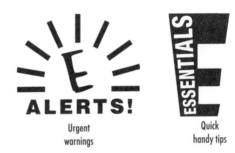

## ALERTS!

Urgent
warnings

## ESSENTIALS

Quick
handy tips

## Editorial

Director of Innovation: Paula Munier

Editorial Director: Laura M. Daly

Executive Editor, Series Books: Brielle K. Matson

Associate Copy Chief: Sheila Zwiebel

Acquisitions Editor: Kerry Smith

Associate Development Editor: Elizabeth Kassab

Production Editor: Casey Ebert

## Production

Director of Manufacturing: Susan Beale

Production Project Manager: Michelle Roy Kelly

Prepress: Erick DaCosta, Matt LeBlanc

Design Manager: Heather Blank

Interior Layout: Heather Barrett,
Brewster Brownville, Colleen Cunningham

Visit the entire Everything® series at www.everything.com

# THE EVERYTHING®

# CALORIE COUNTING COOKBOOK

Eat great and lose weight by calculating
your daily calories, fat, carbs, and fiber

Paula Conway

Technical Review by Brierley E. Wright, R.D.

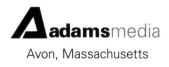

Avon, Massachusetts

*To my mother, my husband, and my babies with four feet and paws.*

An Everything® Series Book.
Everything® and everything.com® are registered trademarks of F+W Publications, Inc.

Published by Adams Media, an F+W Publications Company
57 Littlefield Street, Avon, MA 02322 U.S.A.
*www.adamsmedia.com*

ISBN 10: 1-59869-416-2
ISBN 13: 978-1-59869-416-1

Printed in the United States of America.

J I H G F E D C B A

**Library of Congress Cataloging-in-Publication Data**
available from the publisher.

This publication is designed to provide accurate and authoritative information with regard to the subject matter covered. It is sold with the understanding that the publisher is not engaged in rendering legal, accounting, or other professional advice. If legal advice or other expert assistance is required, the services of a competent professional person should be sought.

—From a *Declaration of Principles* jointly adopted by a Committee of the American Bar Association and a Committee of Publishers and Associations

Many of the designations used by manufacturers and sellers to distinguish their products are claimed as trademarks. Where those designations appear in this book and Adams Media was aware of a trademark claim, the designations have been printed with initial capital letters.

*This book is available at quantity discounts for bulk purchases.*
*For information, please call 1-800-289-0963.*

# Contents

# Acknowledgments

To my mother for helping me write this book every single step of the way; to my outstanding agent, Lori Perkins, for tremendous vision and hard work; to my genius husband who continues to stay up late after a long day's work to help me get things done, and never complains; to my puppy, Marley, who makes me walk him for at least two hours every day to make sure I keep my body in check; and to Delores for taking care of all the animals when I travel.

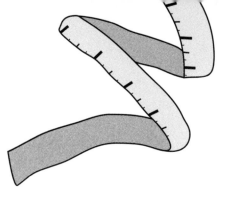

# Introduction

Preparing meals that are both satisfying and low in calories is easier than you think. Based on a 1,200- to 1,500-calorie-a-day diet, *The Everything® Calorie Counting Cookbook* does the work for you, and what could be better than that? Let's face it, what we all really want is simplicity—fast and easy dishes that taste great and keep the weight off. This book delivers just that in an easy-to-follow format.

Breakfasts are broken down into four simple categories: eggs and omelets; French toast, waffles and pancakes; smoothies and shakes; and breads and muffins. Effortless entrees include meat, fish, fowl, and vegetarian options. Appetizers, dips, and soups are included along with chapters for salads, dressings, and sandwiches and wraps. Low-calorie snacks and decadent, trouble-free desserts make this the most undemanding calorie-counting cookbook you'll ever find.

In each chapter you will find ways to reduce calories and fat content in your foods and recipes by cooking with seasonings to add flavor instead of fat. As you journey through this book, you will find some wonderful recipes, many passed down from generations that have been dressed up over the years to make preparing each meal a stimulating experience. For example, Toad in a Hole is an old-time family favorite breakfast. It's a simple piece of toast with a circle cut out of the center and a fried or baked egg in the middle. It's fun to look at, fun to make, and with some added spices, sausage, and seasonings it takes on a whole new exciting flavor.

Conway Welsh Rarebit Melt is a family recipe from the Middle Ages and beginning of the Renaissance. Nifty ingredients like light beer and Tabasco make this rarebit pop. The Vancho Chicken Paprikas was handed down from my Slovakian great-grandmother, prepared with bursts of flavor from paprika, lemon, and tomato. John's Turkey Chili is thick and meaty, perfect for rainy or winter days and football games, without a lot of fat and calories. The honey cakes and baked apples will astonish; they are sweet and savory, and lower in calories.

There are also some great appetizers and snacks like the cheese lace, which is prepared with simple fanfare by baking finely sliced cubes of low-fat cheese until crispy. Sprinkled with seasonings or parmesan, this entertaining favorite is simply addictive. Whatever your individual tastes or cravings, there are many tasty options inside this book. Happy eating!

# 1

# Counting Calories

Losing weight can be an overwhelming pro-posal, but here's some great news: if you main-tain a 1,200- to 1,500-calorie-a-day regimen, you can eat just about anything. Weight loss always comes down to your daily caloric intake and out-put. If you consume fewer calories than you burn, you will lose weight. In this cookbook you will find some new meals that you can create to achieve your weight-loss goals without giving anything up or sacrificing taste. Simply put, you can have your cake and eat it too!

# Calorie Counting 101

Nutritionists, dieticians, and healthcare professionals agree that healthy eating includes counting calories and sticking to a low-fat diet. These basics are essential for long-term healthy weight loss. Losing weight by counting calories helps to build your knowledge and awareness of how many calories your body needs to function and what is in the foods you consume. Counting calories does not take a lot of time or effort; it's flexible enough to fit into most lifestyles and can accommodate personal preferences. Dieting by counting calories means there are no forbidden foods.

## How Many Calories Does It Take?

A calorie is a unit of energy associated with food and dieting. A calorie is defined as the amount of energy, or heat, required to raise the temperature of 1 gram of water 1°C. It is in effect the amount of potential energy that a food contains. The body uses this energy to live and breathe.

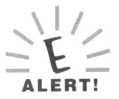

It is crucial to check with your doctor before beginning any weight-loss regimen, especially if it includes physical activity your body is not used to. Your doctor may have suggestions for how to proceed with your plan and can help you establish your goals.

To lose weight, the amount of calories you consume must be less than the amount of calories you burn off during the day. Any calories your body does not burn are converted to fat. The amount of calories your body needs varies depending on your body type and size and the amount of energy you spend in a given day. For weight loss, consuming 1,200 to 1,500 calories a day is recommended for most people, but if you're very physically active you may need a few hundred more calories to fuel your system. The general rule is to eat 300 to 500 calories less than you need each day to lose weight. This may translate into losing one to two pounds per week. Losing weight and keeping it off is about making a change in lifestyle; it is better to lose slowly than to drop large amounts quickly that you can't keep off.

## The Food Pyramid

In 2005, the U.S. Department of Agriculture unveiled a new model of its decade-old food pyramid. The new model, available at *www.mypyramid.gov*, allows you to personalize your own pyramid based on age, gender, height, weight, and activity level. A related tool, the MyPyramid Tracker (*www .mypyramidtracker.gov*), provides an in-depth analysis of your diet and exercise routine and allows you to record your daily activities and food intake.

You can use the new pyramid to balance your diet. Figure out what foods you should have most of and incorporate them into your diet. Physical activity is also an important part of losing weight and keeping it off.

## What Is a Healthy Diet?

A healthy diet is a well-balanced diet, and a well-balanced diet is important because it has a direct effect on your health. You want the right carbohydrates, high in fiber, water, vitamins, and minerals. Fruits, vegetables, grains, and legumes should make up the bulk of the calories you consume. They are high in complex carbohydrates, fiber, vitamins, and minerals, low in fat, and free of cholesterol. The rest of your calories should come from low-fat dairy products, lean meat and poultry, and fish.

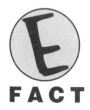

**FACT**

Read nutrition labels. New labels require food companies to list trans fats on the labels to allow consumers to track how much they eat. Trans fats are a form of hydrogenated oil that has been linked to increased risk of heart disease. Some restaurants include nutrition information on their menus; this makes it simple for you to find healthy options when you eat out.

## Desserts and Snacks

The more active you are, the more you can treat yourself to sweets. As long as your overall diet is low in fat and rich in complex carbohydrates, there is nothing wrong with an occasional cheeseburger or some ice cream. Just be sure to limit the frequency and the portion size. View healthy eating as an opportunity to expand your range of choices by trying foods—especially vegetables, grains, or fruits—that you don't normally eat. A healthy diet doesn't have to mean eating bland or unappealing foods.

## Your Calorie-Counting Plan

You can start your calorie-counting plan simply by using just a few steps to keep track of your progress.

- **Audit your habits.** Start with a food journal. It will allow you to take a close look at what you're eating and drinking and identify where you can make changes.
- **Stock up on fruits and vegetables.** Fruits and vegetables are generally low in calories and they are high in vitamin, mineral, and fiber content. They give you the satisfaction of feeling full. The USDA recommends seven to nine servings of fruits and vegetables each day.
- **Take it with you.** Take wholesome foods with you wherever you go so you're not tempted to hit the fast-food drive-through or the vending machines at work. Fruits, vegetables, nonfat yogurt, whole grain cereals, bread, and dried fruit will allow you to snack throughout the day and not feel hungry.
- **Make small changes.** There's nothing groundbreaking about making small changes, but it's the best way to start a new eating plan without feeling overwhelmed. Cut back on portions, downsize your plate, and add new foods in small increments.
- **Bring on the cheerleaders.** Surround yourself with people who will encourage you. Getting support from people who have been through or understand your goals is a great way to learn and boost your confidence.
- **Use a food scale.** Calories are measured in weight, so the best way to keep track of how many calories you eat is to invest in a small food scale to weigh your portions and ingredients.

Make calorie counting work for you by keeping track of your food and activities, eating healthy foods, and staying motivated. Make sure your body gets the nutrients it requires every day. It may take some adjustment for you, but start slowly and stick with it. Don't expect to see your weight drop instantly; it may take some time for your body to react to changes in diet and exercise.

# Fat Facts

Fats come directly from the food we eat and are broken down in the digestive system by an enzyme called lipase before being transported in the blood stream. Both muscle and fat cells absorb the digested fats and either burn the fat through activity or store it for later use. The fact is, however, that humans need fat as part of a healthy diet. Essential fatty acids must be obtained from food because the body has no way of producing them internally.

## Fat for Energy

Certain vitamins (vitamins A, D, E, and K) are fat soluble, and eating fat is the only way to get these vitamins into the body. Fat contains twice as many calories per gram as either proteins or carbohydrates, which makes fats an excellent source of energy. This is fine—as long as that energy is used.

## Fat in the Body

Fat is found in several places throughout the body. The majority is stored just under the skin. The thickness of the fat under the skin varies from body area to body area. It tends to be thickest at the waist, and is practically nonexistent at the eyelids. Fat is stored to be used when food is not being eaten and provides energy required for exercise.

# Maximize Your Weight Loss

There are all sorts of lifestyle adjustments you can make that will jolt your metabolism to help you increase the amount of calories you burn.

## Don't Miss Breakfast

You never, ever want to miss breakfast—or any meals for that matter—because this can lead the body to function in starvation mode, which ultimately slows your metabolic rate and can cause you to eat more later on in the day; it's a lose-lose proposition. Evening out the calories throughout the day will make you less hungry, which makes you less likely to binge.

## Satiate to Lose Weight

Water and water-based foods like fruits and vegetables may help suppress your appetite so you feel full. Lean proteins like fish and chicken also help satiate the appetite so you eat less while feeling full. Eat fish and chicken for your meals, and stock up on healthy snacks so you won't be tempted to go for junk food.

**ESSENTIAL**

Exercise is an important part of healthy weight loss. Start simple, and make it fun. If you have kids, play tag, ride bikes, or just turn on the radio and dance. Do some window shopping in your local mall to get moving, and use your living room as a workout space by popping in your favorite DVD workout.

## Sleep Well

Sleep loss wreaks havoc with the hormones that regulate hunger and satiety. It's the quality of sleep that makes the difference. Sleeping silently orchestrates a symphony of hormonal activity that is tied to the appetite. Recent studies show that two hormones, leptin and ghrelin, help control appetite. When you sleep well, leptin levels are higher and leptin sends a signal to the brain that you are full. Conversely, if your sleep is disrupted, ghrelin is produced in higher quantity and this sends a signal to the brain that you are hungry. If you are well rested—a typical person needs seven to nine hours of sleep per night—your metabolism will thank you.

# Your Personal Coach

Exercise is important when counting calories, but you can aim too high and fall fast. Avoiding some common exercise mistakes will help you succeed.

- **Check with your doctor.** Before you begin an exercise regimen make sure your body is in condition to take on new levels of activity.
- **Don't take on too much too soon.** A gradual introduction to exercise, especially if you haven't been exercising up to this point, is best. Don't sign up for advanced aerobics just because you've decided that today is the day to start exercising. Instead, try 30 minutes of walking every other day and work up to the heavier workouts.
- **Exercise with a goal in mind.** Today you might walk for 30 minutes, but tomorrow you'll add another 15 minutes by taking a detour to a friend's house or favorite park while walking your dog. Selecting four or five short-term goals will make you more successful in the end.
- **Use the right gear.** We don't sleep in our sneakers and we don't run in our slippers. If you don't have proper walking or working-out gear you can ultimately do more damage to your body and sabotage your plans. You don't always need to spend a lot of money, but it's important not to skimp on some things like a good pair of running shoes.
- **Lift weights.** You can start out with two-pound weights and work your way up. Lifting weights helps build muscle and speeds up your metabolic rate. To ensure the proper weight-lifting technique and your own safety, get an introduction from a professional at your local gym.
- **Don't compare yourself to others.** The focus is you, not the world around you. People come in all shapes and sizes, and everyone improves in different ways.

Adults should get at least 30 minutes of exercise per day, and you may have to work up to more to lose weight. Vary your exercise routine and incorporate new activities to keep your mind and your body interested.

# Supermarket Smarts

Getting into the groove of counting calories will make the supermarket an entirely different place. For example, you can still enjoy a plate of pancakes, but you'll need to look for the best mixes and syrups within your calorie range. Look for great low-calorie options without added sugar: Aunt Jemima Lite Syrup has 100 calories per serving, yet Log Cabin Sugar-Free Syrup has only 35 calories per serving. Making the right choice involves reading the labels carefully to determine which is best for you. Here are some simple supermarket shopping tips:

- **Soy vs. Dairy.** Soy-based foods supply nutrition but are not essential for your body's health. The number of calories and amount of calcium and vitamin D in fat-free milk and light soy milk are similar. Ultimately the decision is up to you.
- **Butter vs. Margarine.** If you want to avoid trans fat, choose butter over margarine. Either way you go, use them sparingly. You could also opt for something like Smart Balance, a non-butter option that does not contain trans fats.
- **Which eggs are best?** Eggs have more cholesterol than any other food, and nutritionally brown eggs are identical to white eggs. Egg Beaters and other egg substitutes are a nutritious option. They use the egg whites and leave out the yolk, the primary source of cholesterol.
- **Which oil is best?** Olive oil is actually no healthier than most other cooking oils. When choosing oils for cooking or salad dressings, your main health consideration should be avoiding hydrogenated oils because of their high levels of trans fat. Whether your oil comes from soybeans, safflower seeds, corn, nuts, or olives, they are all high in calories—120 per tablespoon—so use them sparingly.
- **Candy, cookies, and chips.** Here's where you simply need to choose wisely. Instead of potato chips drenched in saturated fats and oils, go for baked chips and salsa. Instead of double-stuff Oreos, try chocolate sticks dipped in light whipped cream. You can still enjoy sweet treats, but scale back on them and opt for lower-calorie alternatives.

# Eating Out Strategies

When you're eating out or buying food that has been prepared for you, it's easy to consume too much fat, salt, and calories. You can also end up eating more than you would have done if you had made the food yourself. The simplest tip, but not always the easiest, is to remember that you don't need to clear your plate. Eat slowly and stop when you're full.

Here are some eating out tips:

- Don't eat before you arrive.
- Drink water. Calories sneak into your diet through the beverages you drink. Wine, beer, mixed drinks, soft drinks, coffee, tea, and even juice can easily increase your daily caloric intake by a few hundred calories.
- Share the appetizer or dessert with a friend. If there is a dessert on the menu you really want, skip the appetizer.
- When you're ordering a variety of dishes, for example in a tapas bar or restaurant, be careful not to order too many.
- If your meal doesn't come with vegetables, order some as a side dish or have a salad with your meal.
- Wait until you've eaten your main course before you order a dessert. By the time you finish your entrée, you may be too full to enjoy a dessert.
- If you want a healthy dessert, go for fresh fruit or sorbet.

Just because the nutritional information isn't right in front of you doesn't mean you can order whatever you want. Learn to zero in on healthy options on the menu. Look at the cooking technique. "Fried" translates into more oil—you can do better. Go for a grilled entrée instead.

In the end, it doesn't matter whether you eat out or eat in. As long as you keep track of the calories you eat, stick to a healthy diet, and exercise regularly, you will be on the path to healthy weight control.

# 2

# Eggs and Omelets

# Eggs Benedict

To add some crunch, toast the bread before serving.

*Yields 4 servings*
Calories: 295
Fat: 20 grams
Protein: 13 grams
Carbohydrates: 16 grams
Cholesterol: 241 milligrams

*3 tablespoons skim milk*
*½ cup low-fat mayonnaise*
*4 eggs*
*4 slices bacon*
*4 slices whole wheat bread or 2*
  *whole wheat English muffins*

1. Mix the skim milk with the mayonnaise and heat in the microwave for about 40 seconds to warm.

2. Crack each egg into individual microwaveable bowls, being careful not to break the yolks.

3. Cover each bowl with plastic wrap and microware on high until the whites are cooked and yolks firm, about 2 minutes.

4. In a skillet, cook the bacon.

5. Place the bacon on the whole wheat bread slices.

6. Add the eggs on the bacon and top each egg with 2 tablespoons of mayonnaise mixture.

# Egg and Cheese Breakfast Pizza

You can also add chunks of beef fillets, ham, or mushrooms to give this pizza more pizzazz.

*Yields 8 servings*
Calories: 189
Fat: 3 grams
Protein: 9 grams
Carbohydrates: 30 grams
Cholesterol: 4 milligrams

*1 tablespoon all-purpose flour*
*16-ounce frozen pizza dough*
*cooking spray*
*1½ cups Egg Beaters*
*½ cup fat-free milk*
*½ cup low-fat cheese, any flavor*

1. Preheat oven to 375°F.

2. Sprinkle flour on a flat surface and roll out the pizza dough to a 12" circle, building up the edges so they're thick and high. Place the dough on a nonstick baking sheet and then prick the dough thoroughly with a fork.

3. Bake until light brown, about 15 minutes.

4. While the crust is baking, coat a skillet with cooking spray and beat the Egg Beaters and milk in a large bowl.

5. Scramble the mixture over medium heat, then place scrambled eggs on pizza crust and sprinkle with cheese.

6. Bake 7 minutes to melt the cheese, then slice with knife or pizza roller.

# Baked Scrambled Eggs

*Baked scrambled eggs are best when served immediately from the oven.*

1. Preheat oven to 350°F.

2. In a glass measuring cup, heat the butter in the microwave until melted.

3. In a separate bowl whisk the eggs, salt, and milk.

4. Pour the melted butter and then the eggs into a 9" x 13" baking dish.

5. Bake uncovered for 8 minutes, then stir and add cheese if desired. Bake for 10 to 15 more minutes or until eggs are set.

## Incredible Edible Eggs

Eggs provide a tremendous amount of protein and very little carbohydrates, and they make you feel full. You should have one egg a day, but remember that so many things we consume daily already contain eggs. Before you have your daily dose of egg, make sure your other meals and snacks do not contain egg or you could overdo it.

*Yields 12 servings*
Calories: 213
Fat: 16 grams
Protein: 13 grams
Carbohydrates: 3 grams
Cholesterol: 374 milligrams

½ cup butter
20 eggs
2 teaspoons salt
1¾ cups fat-free milk
½ cup shredded low-fat cheese (optional)

# Simple and Skinny Cheese Omelet

*For an even skinnier omelet, use fat-free cheese.*

*Yields 2 servings*
Calories: 129
Fat: 7 grams
Protein: 14 grams
Carbohydrates: 2 grams
Cholesterol: 15 milligrams

*½ cup fat-free Egg Beaters*
*1 teaspoon olive oil*
*½ cup low-fat shredded cheese*

1. Heat the olive oil in a small skillet on low heat, then pour the Egg Beaters in to coat the surface and cook until edges show firmness.

2. Sprinkle the cheese evenly over the egg mixture and fold one side over the other.

3. Flip the half-moon omelet so both sides are evenly cooked.

# Mary's Low-Fat Egg and Spinach Cupcakes

*Top these cupcakes with a slice of tomato and sprinkle on some shredded cheese to add a nice touch of color and great flavor.*

*Yields 5 servings*
Calories: 175
Fat: 10 grams
Protein: 16 grams
Carbohydrates: 5 grams
Cholesterol: 113 milligrams

*10 ounces chopped frozen spinach*
*2 eggs*
*1 cup skim ricotta cheese*
*1 cup low-fat shredded mozzarella cheese*

1. Preheat oven to 350°F.

2. Place cupcake liners in 12-hole cupcake tin.

3. Heat spinach in microwave until soft and warm.

4. Whip the eggs and add the spinach. Blend together.

5. Fold in the ricotta and shredded cheese.

6. Fill each cup with egg-spinach mixture, about ½" per cup.

7. Bake 30–35 minutes.

# Barely There Egg White Bruschetta

Add two more slices of bread to spread out the bruschetta if you want to serve more people.

1. Beat egg whites and eggs together.

2. Heat chopped tomato, mushroom, and onion in a large skillet. Add egg mixture and scramble. Add basil, salt, and pepper as you scramble.

3. Toast bread and top with the egg mixture.

### Eggs and Cholesterol

Eggs are the leading source of cholesterol in American diets. To keep your cholesterol levels in check, try to stick to one egg or one egg yolk and two egg whites per day. Purchase eggs from chickens raised on a vegetarian diet rather than animal fats and animal by-products.

*Yields 2 servings*
Calories: 395
Fat: 13 grams
Protein: 34 grams
Carbohydrates: 39 grams
Cholesterol: 425 milligrams

*7 egg whites*
*4 whole eggs*
*1 chopped tomato*
*½ cup chopped mushrooms*
*1 small onion*
*¼ cup fresh basil*
*½ teaspoon salt*
*½ teaspoon pepper*
*4 slices whole grain bread*

# Eggs Florentine

You can replace the mayonnaise with nonfat yogurt.
This recipe is particularly good with nonfat vanilla yogurt.

1. Preheat oven to 350°F. Place muffins on a baking sheet.

2. Crack an egg onto each muffin. Bake for 10 minutes.

3. Meanwhile, heat the spinach in the microwave until soft and warm, about two minutes.

4. Add low-fat mayonnaise, salt, and pepper to spinach. Blend together.

5. Remove muffins and top with the spinach mixture. Add a teaspoon of shredded cheese and serve.

*Yields 2 servings*
Calories: 260
Fat: 10 grams
Protein: 15 grams
Carbohydrates: 31 grams
Cholesterol: 217 milligrams

*2 English muffins*
*2 eggs*
*5 ounces chopped frozen spinach*
*1 tablespoon low-fat mayonnaise*
*1 teaspoon salt*
*1 teaspoon pepper*
*2 teaspoons shredded low-fat cheese*

# Toad in a Hole

*Yields 2 servings*
Calories: 72
Fat: 3 grams
Protein: 5 grams
Carbohydrates: 7 grams
Cholesterol: 106 milligrams

1 slice bread, any kind
nonfat cooking spray
1 egg

In Britain, Toad in a Hole involves baking sausages and Yorkshire pudding in a large pan with bacon fat drippings and flour, but this recipe— a Pennsylvania Dutch favorite—is far simpler and far less fattening.

1. Use a circular cookie cutter to cut a hole in the center of a slice of bread.

2. Place on a warm skillet, sprayed lightly with nonfat cooking spray.

3. Crack the egg and put it in the hole in the bread.

4. Fry and flip to desired consistency.

5. Salt and pepper to taste.

## Flipping Toads

As it cooks, the egg adheres to the bread. This makes it super simple to flip the bread in the pan without worrying about dislodging the egg. Be sure to flip your eggs after they've had time to set. Otherwise, you risk getting runny egg all over the place, which won't affect taste but will leave you with a mess.

# Chive and Cheese Omelet

Chives are an excellent herb because they can be purchased
year-round and will keep in the freezer for long periods of time.

1. Beat the egg whites and egg in a small bowl. Mix in the salt.

2. Heat the olive oil in a small skillet on low heat.

3. Pour the egg mixture in to coat the surface.

4. Cook until edges show firmness.

5. Sprinkle the cheese evenly over the egg mixture, then do the same with the chives. Fold one side over the other.

6. Flip the half-moon omelet so both sides are evenly cooked.

## Perfect Omelets

A classic omelet should be very fluffy and has to be eaten immediately; it's delicate and ethereal. The fantastic thing about omelets is that you can stuff them with all kinds of things. Various veggies, fruits, and cheeses make exciting omelets. Try mixing some cheddar cheese sauce and broccoli or some Brie and raspberries for your next omelet and enjoy the flavors!

*Yields 2 servings*
Calories: 156
Fat: 11 grams
Protein: 14 grams
Carbohydrates: 1.5 grams
Cholesterol: 109 milligrams

4 large egg whites
1 large whole egg
¼ teaspoon salt
1 tablespoon olive oil
¼ cup reduced-fat shredded
    cheddar cheese
2 tablespoons chopped fresh chives

# Sausage and Mushroom Omelet

*If you like a little spice, add a dash of Tabasco sauce to kick up the flavor.*

**Yields 2 servings**
Calories: 266
Fat: 20 grams
Protein: 20 grams
Carbohydrates: 2.5 grams
Cholesterol: 141 milligrams

*4 large egg whites*
*1 large whole egg*
*¼ teaspoon salt*
*1 tablespoon olive oil*
*½ cup chopped turkey sausage*
*½ cup chopped mushrooms*

1. Beat the egg whites and egg in a small bowl. Mix in the salt.

2. Heat the olive oil in a small skillet on low heat.

3. Pour the egg mixture in to coat the surface.

4. Cook until edges show firmness.

5. Add the sausage and mushrooms so that they cover the entire mixture evenly. Fold one side over the other.

6. Flip the half moon omelet so both sides are evenly cooked.

# Mama's Mini Mexican Omelet

*If you like pepper, add as much as you like to this recipe. Pepper mixes well with the jalapeño in the cheddar cheese to give this omelet a festive taste.*

1. Beat the egg whites and egg in a small bowl. Mix in the salt.

2. Mix the beans, onions, and shredded cheese gently in a small bowl.

3. Heat the olive oil in a small skillet on low heat.

4. Pour the egg mixture in to coat the surface.

5. Cook until edges show firmness.

6. Add the black beans, chopped onions, and cheese so that they cover the entire egg mixture evenly. Fold one side over the other.

7. Flip the half-moon omelet so both sides are evenly cooked. Serve with salsa.

## Testing Egg Freshness

To test whether an egg is fresh, immerse it in a pan of cool, salted water. If it sinks to the bottom, it is fresh. If it rises to the surface, it is spoiled. If the eggs in your refrigerator are approaching or have passed their freshness date, always perform this test before using the eggs.

---

*Yields 2 servings*
Calories: 245
Fat: 12 grams
Protein: 19 grams
Carbohydrates: 17 grams
Cholesterol: 110 milligrams

*4 large egg whites*
*1 large whole egg*
*¼ teaspoon salt*
*1 tablespoon olive oil*
*½ cup canned black beans, rinsed and drained*
*¼ cup chopped onions*
*1 ounce reduced-fat shredded jalapeño cheddar cheese*
*¼ cup salsa*

# Veggie Egg Beater Omelet

**Yields 2 servings**
Calories: 155
Fat: 8 grams
Protein: 15 grams
Carbohydrates: 9 grams
Cholesterol: 0 milligrams

1 cup Egg Beaters
½ cup water
1 cup chopped tomato
1 cup chopped green peppers
1 tablespoon olive oil

You can buy flavored Egg Beaters, which adds even more taste to an Egg Beater Omelet.

1. Beat the Egg Beaters with water in a small bowl.
2. Mix the chopped tomato and green peppers in a small bowl.
3. Heat the olive oil in a small skillet on low heat.
4. Pour the Egg Beater mixture in to coat the surface.
5. Cook until edges show firmness.
6. Add the vegetable mixture evenly over the eggs. Fold one side over the other.
7. Flip the half-moon omelet so both sides are evenly cooked.

# Very Veggie Chopped Vegetable Omelet

**Yields 2 servings**
Calories: 159
Fat: 10 grams
Protein: 12 grams
Carbohydrates: 8 grams
Cholesterol: 106 milligrams

4 large egg whites
1 large whole egg
¼ teaspoon salt
½ cup chopped red peppers
½ cup chopped green peppers
¼ cup chopped onions
½ cup chopped mushrooms
1 tablespoon olive oil

Vary this recipe by chopping up any vegetable you like
and adding it or substituting it for the peppers.

1. Beat the egg whites and egg in a small bowl. Mix in the salt.
2. Mix the vegetables together in a small bowl.
3. Heat the olive oil in a small skillet on low heat.
4. Pour the egg mixture in to coat the surface.
5. Cook until edges show firmness.
6. Add the vegetable mixture so that it covers the entire egg mixture evenly. Fold one side over the other.
7. Flip the half moon omelet so both sides are evenly cooked.

# Tomato and Spinach Omelet

*If a recipe calls for an egg but does not specify large or small, it does not matter what size you buy. However, if a recipe, like this one, calls for large eggs it is because the recipe needs a larger egg.*

1. Beat the egg whites and egg in a small bowl. Mix in the salt.

2. Heat the spinach in a microwavable bowl for about two minutes or until warm and soft. Mix spinach with chopped tomato.

3. Heat the olive oil in a small skillet on low heat.

4. Pour the egg mixture in to coat the surface.

5. Cook until edges show firmness.

6. Add the spinach and tomato mixture evenly over the eggs. Fold one side over the other.

7. Flip the half-moon omelet so both sides are evenly cooked.

## Leftover Egg Yolks

Stir leftover egg yolks lightly and then freeze them in ice cube trays to be defrosted later to brush on bread as a glaze for baking. Another alternative is to mix them into your dog's food for a shiny coat.

*Yields 2 servings*
Calories: 181
Fat: 10 grams
Protein: 14 grams
Carbohydrates: 10 grams
Cholesterol: 106 milligrams

4 large egg whites
1 large whole egg
¼ teaspoon salt
1 cup cooked frozen spinach
1 cup chopped tomato
1 tablespoon olive oil

# Turkey Omelet with Egg Beaters

*Yields 2 servings*
Calories: 263
Fat: 11 grams
Protein: 34 grams
Carbohydrates: 7 grams
Cholesterol: 53 milligrams

*1 cup Egg Beaters*
*1 cup ground, lean turkey meat*
*½ cup water*
*1 cup chopped tomato*
*1 tablespoon olive oil*

Many people don't think Egg Beaters are real eggs, but they are. They only use the egg white. Vitamins A, B-12, D, and E, along with other nutrients like folic acid and riboflavin are added to preserve what can be lost when the yolk is removed.

1.  Beat the Egg Beaters in a small bowl.

2.  Boil water in a small cooking pot, then add the ground turkey meat until it browns, about five minutes, tossing as it browns.

3.  Mix the chopped tomato with the cooked turkey meat in a small bowl.

4.  Heat the olive oil in a small skillet on low heat.

5.  Pour the Egg Beaters in to coat the surface.

6.  Cook until edges show firmness.

7.  Add the turkey and tomato mixture evenly over the eggs. Fold one side over the other.

8.  Flip the half-moon omelet so both sides are evenly cooked.

# 3

# French Toast, Waffles, and Pancakes

# No-Bulge French Toast

*Yields 2 servings*
Calories: 253
Fat: 8 grams
Protein: 14 grams
Carbohydrates: 34 grams
Cholesterol: 214 milligrams

*2 eggs*
*½ cup skim milk*
*½ teaspoon ground cinnamon*
*½ teaspoon vanilla extract*
*1 tablespoon powdered sugar*
*4 slices bread*

This recipe is great when served with sliced pears or peaches on the side. To sweeten it further you can drizzle a tablespoon of sugar-free maple syrup across the top.

1. Preheat oven to 400°F.

2. Beat eggs and skim milk lightly in a bowl. Add the cinnamon, vanilla, and sugar.

3. Soak the bread in the egg mixture and place on a nonstick baking sheet.

4. Bake for about 10 minutes or until golden.

# Belgian Waffles

*Yields 6–8 servings*
Calories: 246
Fat: 6 grams
Protein: 5 grams
Carbohydrates: 43 grams
Cholesterol: 27 milligrams

*2 cups buttermilk baking mix*
*1 egg, beaten*
*3 tablespoons vegetable oil*
*1½ cups club soda*

You can top these with any fruit you love, like strawberries or blueberries.

1. Preheat waffle maker.

2. Combine baking mix, egg, oil, and club soda in a medium bowl.

3. Fill waffle maker according to baking mix directions. Bake until light and crispy.

## Using Waffle Makers

Rub a little bit of the vegetable oil or nonstick cooking spray on the waffle maker to make sure your waffles come out light and fluffy, never dry. Some historians speculate that ancient Greeks ate primitive waffles, cooked between two hot slabs of metal. Medieval Europeans improved upon the technique and developed the trademark patterned plates we use today.

# Strawberry Waffles

*You can top these with sugar-free Cool Whip and fresh fruit.*

1. Mix egg whites, milk, oat bran, flour, baking powder, and oil in a bowl.

2. Fold strawberries in. Pour batter onto a waffle iron.

3. Bake each batch about 5 minutes or until light and crispy.

## Sweet Scent

The best thing about this recipe—other than the taste, of course—is the delicious aroma that fills the house. It is particularly wonderful on cold winter mornings. It's sure to tickle the noses of those family members who are still in bed.

*Yields 4 servings*
Calories: 348
Fat: 13 grams
Protein: 15 grams
Carbohydrates: 46 grams
Cholesterol: 3 milligrams

*4 egg whites*
*2 cups skim milk*
*1 cup oat bran cereal*
*1 cup self-rising flour*
*1 teaspoon baking powder*
*3 tablespoons vegetable oil*
*1 cup chopped strawberries*

# Stuffed French Toast

*Use up more calories for breakfast and cut a thick slice of bread.*
*The stuffing is easier and you'll get a great big stuffed French toast.*

1. Prepare a skillet with the butter-flavored spray.

2. Slice French bread into 1"-thick slices.

3. Cut a pocket through the top of each slice, ¾ of the way through the bread.

4. Insert cream cheese and preserve.

5. Combine milk, vanilla, cinnamon, and nutmeg to make the batter.

6. Dip the bread in the batter and cook on the skillet.

## Soaking Bread

The fresher your bread, the more it falls apart in the batter. Use bread that is nearing the end of its shelf life. It will be a little tougher and will hold together better when soaked in batter.

*Yields 4 servings*
Calories: 319
Fat: 4 grams
Protein: 11 grams
Carbohydrates: 58 grams
Cholesterol: 4 milligrams

*butter-flavored cooking spray*
*4 slices French bread*
*4 teaspoons reduced-fat cream cheese*
*4 teaspoons favorite preserve*
*1 cup skim milk divided into 4 servings*
*1 teaspoon vanilla*
*1 teaspoon cinnamon or to taste*
*½ teaspoon nutmeg or to taste*

# No-Bulge Blueberry French Toast à la Mode

_Yields 6 servings_
Calories: 289
Fat: 3 grams
Protein: 17 grams
Carbohydrates: 50 grams
Cholesterol: 2 milligrams

_14 slices bread_
_¾ cup blueberries_
_1½ cups fat-free Egg Beaters_
_2 cups skim milk_
_2 teaspoons vanilla extract_
_1 teaspoon ground cinnamon_
_2 tablespoons powdered sugar_

_Add ¼ cup of some fat-free ice cream to each serving to make it à la mode._

1. Preheat oven to 400°F.

2. Arrange 7 slices of bread in the bottom of a baking dish.

3. Sprinkle the cup of blueberries over the bread, spreading them out evenly.

4. Whisk the milk, Egg Beaters, ground cinnamon, and vanilla in a bowl.

5. Pour half of the milk mixture over the blueberries and bread, then top with the remaining bread slices and pour leftover milk mixture atop this.

6. Cover the dish with aluminum foil and bake for 20 minutes. Uncover the dish and bake until the top is a nice golden brown.

7. After baking, sprinkle with the powdered sugar and then slice into six servings.

### Top It Off
Peaches, pears, and cherries are good fruit fillings for this recipe. Whatever fruit you love best can be used. Buy fruit that's in season at your local market or use leftovers from fruit-picking expeditions.

# Apple Yogurt Cinnamon Pancakes

You can substitute ½ cup berries for the apples.

1. Combine the egg, yogurt, and oil in a blender until smooth.

2. Sift the flour, sugar, baking powder, baking soda, cinnamon, and salt together. Add to yogurt mixture and blend.

3. Prepare a hot griddle with the butter spray.

4. Ladle about ⅛ cup of the mixture onto the griddle.

5. Sprinkle each of the pancakes with apples and cook until bubbles form in the pancake. Flip over and cook until done.

## Blender Pancakes

These pancakes are super light and super easy to make in the blender. You can add the cinnamon to the ingredients or roll the apple slices in the cinnamon to coat them.

*Yields 4 servings*
Calories: 245
Fat: 6 grams
Protein: 8 grams
Carbohydrates: 35 grams
Cholesterol: 57 milligrams

*1 egg*
*1 cup plain fat-free yogurt*
*1 tablespoon canola oil*
*1 cup flour*
*1 tablespoon sugar*
*1 teaspoon baking powder*
*½ teaspoon baking soda*
*1 teaspoon cinnamon*
*pinch of salt*
*butter-flavored cooking spray*
*½ cup thinly sliced apple*

# Creamy Fruit-Topped Waffles

This is a very special recipe because it is entirely homemade and will keep friends and family alike coming back for more. The finer you chop your fruit, the tastier the waffle.

1. Combine all ingredients except fruit and cream in a blender until smooth.

2. Mix sliced fruit with heavy cream in separate bowl.

3. Pour batter onto the waffle maker.

4. Once cooked, top with the creamy fruit topping.

## Adding Oatmeal

The dry oatmeal gives this recipe a nice texture. You can also add flavored oatmeal to increase the flavor. The fruit sweetens the meal, but eat the waffles quickly before the fruit topping has time to make them soggy.

*Yields 2 servings*
Calories: 281
Fat: 8 grams
Protein: 16 grams
Carbohydrates: 38 grams
Cholesterol: 23 milligrams

*½ cup dry oatmeal*
*½ cup nonfat cottage cheese*
*3 egg whites*
*2 tablespoons Splenda*
*1 teaspoon cinnamon*
*1 teaspoon vanilla*
*1 sliced banana*
*½ cup sliced strawberries*
*2 tablespoons heavy cream*

# Banana Chocolate Chip Pancake Wrap

**Yields 2 servings**
Calories: 318
Fat: 8 grams
Protein: 16 grams
Carbohydrates: 48 grams
Cholesterol: 3 milligrams

½ cup dry oatmeal
½ cup nonfat cottage cheese
3 egg whites
2 tablespoons Splenda
1 teaspoon cinnamon
1 teaspoon vanilla
1 banana
¼ cup of semi-sweet chocolate
chips

The chocolate chips sweeten this pancake recipe and are best when applied immediately after you take the pancakes off the griddle so they start to melt into the pancakes.

1. Combine oatmeal, cottage cheese, egg whites, Splenda, cinnamon, and vanilla in a blender until smooth.

2. Mash banana in a bowl.

3. Fold mashed bananas in with pancake mix.

4. Pour four individual pancakes on griddle, poured thinly.

5. Remove from griddle and place a few chocolate chips on each pancake. Fold over like a cigar.

# Ginger-Pear Wheat Pancakes

**Yields 3 servings**
Calories: 267
Fat: 1 gram
Protein: 9 grams
Carbohydrates: 60 grams
Cholesterol: 0 milligrams

1½ cups whole wheat flour
2 tablespoons applesauce
1 tablespoon brown sugar
1 cup water
1½ teaspoons baking powder
1½ teaspoons ground ginger
1 teaspoon ground cinnamon
2 chopped pears

Add ¼ cup of chopped walnuts to the chopped pears to give these a little texture and kick.

1. Combine the whole wheat flour, applesauce, brown sugar, water, and baking powder in a medium bowl.

2. Add the ginger and ground cinnamon.

3. Fold in the chopped pears.

4. Pour the batter onto a hot griddle or skillet, ¼ cup for each pancake, and cook until golden.

The Everything Calorie Counting Cookbook

# Oatmeal and Buttermilk Pancakes

*Diabetics can substitute Splenda for sugar. It tastes the same and keeps it a sugar-free meal.*

1. Combine oat bran, flour, sugar, baking powder, baking soda, and salt in a bowl.

2. Whisk together buttermilk and Egg Beaters in a small bowl. Pour mixture over dry ingredients and stir together until just blended.

3. Prepare a hot griddle with butter-flavored spray. Pour ¼ cup pancake batter on the griddle. Cook until bubbles appear and edges are brown. Flip and cook until done.

**_Yields 6 servings_**
Calories: 158
Fat: 2 grams
Protein: 7 grams
Carbohydrates: 29 grams
Cholesterol: 3 milligrams

*1 cup uncooked oatmeal*
*½ cup flour*
*¼ cup sugar*
*1 teaspoon baking powder*
*1 teaspoon baking soda*
*⅛ teaspoon salt*
*2 cups low-fat buttermilk*
*¼ cup Egg Beaters*
*butter-flavored spray*

# Whole Grain Pancakes with Blackberry Syrup

*Serve these pancakes when you have guests for a big brunch.*

1. Sift the flour, milk powder, baking powder, baking soda, and salt in a large bowl.

2. Stir in the whole wheat flour.

3. Combine Splenda, eggs, water, butter, and vinegar in a small bowl.

4. Pour this egg mixture in with the flour mixture and mix until smooth.

5. Mix blackberries and heavy cream in blender until smooth and creamy.

6. In a frying pan or griddle, pour about ¼ cup batter for each pancake and cook until golden.

7. Serve with sliced banana and blackberry topping.

**_Yields 12 servings_**
Calories: 266
Fat: 11 grams
Protein: 10 grams
Carbohydrates: 34 grams
Cholesterol: 98 milligrams

*1⅓ cup whole dry milk powder*
*1 cup all-purpose flour*
*1 teaspoon baking powder*
*1 teaspoon baking soda*
*1 teaspoon salt*
*2 cups whole wheat flour*
*¾ cup Splenda*
*4 eggs*
*3 cups water*
*¼ cup butter*
*3 tablespoons white vinegar*
*1 cup blackberries*
*2 tablespoons heavy cream*
*1 sliced banana*

# Baked Gingerbread Pancakes

*Yields 4 servings*
Calories: 188
Fat: <1 gram
Protein: 13 grams
Carbohydrates: 33 grams
Cholesterol: 1 milligram

*butter-flavored cooking spray*
*½ cup fat-free milk*
*½ cup flour*
*½ cup unsweetened applesauce*
*1 cup Egg Beaters*
*1 tablespoon dark molasses*
*2 tablespoons Splenda*
*½ teaspoon ground ginger*
*½ teaspoon ground cinnamon*
*¼ teaspoon salt*
*1 cup nonfat vanilla yogurt*

*This puffy cake-like mixture will deflate as soon as you remove it from the oven. Do not be alarmed, it's supposed to do that. You can use any flavor of nonfat yogurt if you want to alter the taste slightly.*

1. Preheat oven to 425°F.

2. Coat a circular cake pan with butter-flavored cooking spray.

3. Stir all ingredients except yogurt in a medium bowl and whisk until batter is smooth.

4. Pour batter onto cake pan and bake until it puffs up, about 15 minutes.

5. Cut into 4 slices like a pizza and serve.

6. Top each slice with about ¼ cup of the yogurt

# Banana Three-Grain Pancakes

*Serves 4–6*
Calories: 225
Fat: 3 grams
Protein: 11 grams
Carbohydrates: 40 grams
Cholesterol: 56 milligrams

*⅓ cup sifted all-purpose flour*
*⅔ cup whole wheat flour*
*⅔ cup uncooked rolled oats*
*pinch of salt*
*1 teaspoon baking powder*
*1 tablespoon Splenda*
*1 cup nonfat buttermilk*
*1 egg*
*2 egg whites*
*½ banana*
*butter-flavored cooking spray*

*Serve these hearty pancakes with a dollop of unsweetened applesauce and a dash of cinnamon.*

1. Combine the whole wheat flour, all-purpose flour, rolled oats, baking powder, salt, and Splenda in a bowl.

2. Add the buttermilk, egg, and egg whites and mix until blended. Slice the banana and fold into mixture. Leave for 5 minutes.

3. Spray a hot griddle with cooking spray.

4. Pour ¼ cup of batter onto the griddle for each pancake and cook until bubbles appear in the batter.

5. Turn pancakes and cook on other side until edges brown.

# 4

# Smoothies and Breakfast Shakes

# Banana-Berry

You can replace the yogurt with soy yogurt and the
milk with soy or rice milk if you have a milk allergy.

1. Combine all ingredients in a blender until smooth. Pour into a tall glass.

### Protein Shakes
Give your smoothie an instant protein boost by adding a tablespoon of peanut butter to the smoothie mixture. You can also add protein powder to the smoothie to really pack a punch.

*Yields 1 serving*
Calories: 365
Fat: 2 grams
Protein: 21 grams
Carbohydrates: 71 grams
Cholesterol: 7 milligrams

*1 banana*
*1 cup raspberries*
*1 cup nonfat yogurt*
*½ cup skim milk*

# Blueberry

Using nonfat vanilla yogurt gives any smoothie a rich, vanilla undertone.

1. Combine all ingredients in a blender until smooth. Pour into a tall glass.

### Smoothie History
The smoothie was officially born in California, where smoothie bars are as plentiful as blondes. Its origin has been linked to the Orange Julius of the 1970s or to the Cuban batido, a traditional Cuban tropical fruit milkshake.

*Yields 1 serving*
Calories: 261
Fat: 1 gram
Protein: 19 grams
Carbohydrates: 45 grams
Cholesterol: 7 milligrams

*1 cup blueberries*
*1 cup nonfat yogurt*
*½ cup skim milk*

# Banana-Peach

Add a little low- or nonfat peach or banana yogurt to
get even more flavor out of this delicious smoothie.

1. Combine all ingredients in a blender until smooth. Pour into a tall glass.

## Making Smoothies

Invent your own smoothie by mixing any fruits you desire in a blender with milk and yogurt.
Just keep in mind that if you use a very sour fruit, like a lemon, you should mellow the taste by
balancing it out with something like a banana.

*Yields 1 serving*
Calories: 347
Fat: 1 gram
Protein: 20 grams
Carbohydrates: 67 grams
Cholesterol: 7 milligrams

*1 banana
1 peach, sliced
1 cup nonfat yogurt
½ cup skim milk*

# Blackberry-Apple

When berries are not in season, frozen berries will work just as well.
Frozen berries can also add a nice texture to a berry smoothie. Test the
texture as you blend to get the perfect fruity, crunchy blend.

1. Combine all ingredients in a blender until smooth. Pour into a tall glass.

*Yields 1 serving*
Calories: 380
Fat: 2 grams
Protein: 20 grams
Carbohydrates: 75 grams
Cholesterol: 7 milligrams

*1 cup blackberries
1 apple, sliced
1 cup nonfat yogurt
½ cup skim milk*

# Blackberry-Peach

For an extra sweet pop, add a little honey to the mixture while blending.

1. Combine all ingredients in a blender until smooth. Pour into a tall glass.

### Batch 'Em
Make large batches of smoothies so you can keep single servings in the freezer. Get out a serving as you begin to get ready for your day. This should give the smoothie time to thaw enough for you to stir it when you're ready to have breakfast.

**_Yields 1 serving_**
Calories: 322
Fat: 1 gram
Protein: 20 grams
Carbohydrates: 61 grams
Cholesterol: 7 milligrams

*1 cup blackberries*
*1 large peach, sliced*
*1 cup nonfat yogurt*
*½ cup skim milk*

# Green Tea

This smoothie is great when you add fruit like a peach or banana.

1. Brew 1 cup of green tea, then chill.

2. Combine all ingredients in a blender until smooth. Pour into a tall glass.

### Green Means Good
This smoothie is packed with benefits. Green tea is chock full of antioxidants, which protect living cells from damage and deterioration. Researchers think antioxidants can help prevent cancer and some of the side effects of arthritis.

**_Yields 2 servings_**
Calories: 67
Fat: 0 grams
Protein: 4 grams
Carbohydrates: 13 grams
Cholesterol: 1 milligram

*1 cup brewed green tea, chilled*
*½ cup skim milk*
*½ cup fat-free vanilla ice cream*

# Thick and Sinless Strawberry Smoothie

*This smoothie is thick and creamy, but won't thicken the thighs!*

1. Combine all ingredients in a blender until smooth. Pour into a tall glass.

### Berry Smooth

Use fresh berries for smoothies when they are in season. Half a cup of fresh strawberries contains a great flavor punch and few calories.

*Yields 1 serving*
Calories: 251
Fat: 1 gram
Protein: 15 grams
Carbohydrates: 46 grams
Cholesterol: 5 milligrams

*½ cup fat-free vanilla ice cream*
*1 cup fresh strawberries*
*½ cup nonfat yogurt*
*½ cup skim milk*

# Orange You Ready to Lose Weight? Smoothie

*To add some bulk, add a small orange to the mixture after blending
so you have some sweet orange chunks in the smoothie.*

1. Combine all ingredients in a blender until smooth. Pour into a tall glass.

*Yields 1 serving*
Calories: 221
Fat: 0 grams
Protein: 12 grams
Carbohydrates: 41 grams
Cholesterol: 5 milligrams

*1 cup orange juice*
*½ cup nonfat yogurt*
*½ cup skim milk*

# Fruit Medley

Just like the Green Tea Smoothie, this is a great
option if you're looking to boost your antioxidants.

1. Combine all ingredients in a blender until smooth. Pour into a tall glass.

**Yields 1 serving**

Calories: 272
Fat: 2 grams
Protein: 14 grams
Carbohydrates: 55 grams
Cholesterol: 5 milligrams

¼ cup blueberries
¼ cup fresh strawberries
1 large peach, sliced
1 cup raspberries
½ cup nonfat yogurt
½ cup skim milk

# Calorie-Conscious Carrot Smoothie

The orange and lemon juice sweetens this smoothie so you have
the slimming benefits of carrot with a touch of sweetness.

1. Grate 5 large carrots in a blender or food processor. Separate the grated carrot from the juice using a fine strainer.

2. Blend grated carrot, lemon juice, orange juice, yogurt and skim milk until smooth, then blend in the carrot juice. Pour into a tall glass.

**Yields 1 serving**

Calories: 190
Fat: 1 gram
Protein: 13 grams
Carbohydrates: 34 grams
Cholesterol: 5 milligrams

½ cup finely grated carrots
¼ cup carrot juice
1 tablespoon lemon juice
¼ cup orange juice
½ cup nonfat yogurt
½ cup skim milk

### Carrots

Loaded with beta-carotene, which is essential for healthy eyes, skin, and cell respiration, and has been linked to lower lung and prostate cancer rates, carrots are a nutritious superfood that's cheap and available year-round. Always choose fresh carrots that are crisp and tight-skinned, not limp or marred or covered in brown blemishes.

# Blueberry-Peach

You can top this smoothie with a dollop of sugar-free Cool Whip to make this a delicious dessert.

1. Combine all ingredients in a blender until smooth. Pour into a tall glass.

*Yields 1 serving*
Calories: 220
Fat: 1 gram
Protein: 13 grams
Carbohydrates: 43 grams
Cholesterol: 5 milligrams

½ cup blueberries
1 large peach, sliced
½ cup nonfat yogurt
½ cup skim milk

# Pineapple-Coconut

This pineapple and coconut will transplant you to the Caribbean in minutes. Garnish with a cherry and it's pure bliss.

1. Combine all ingredients in a blender until smooth. Pour into a tall glass.

## Coconut Water

Coconut water is found in young coconuts. It can be drunk straight from the coconut. Contrary to popular belief, coconut milk is not the liquid found inside a whole coconut. It is made from mixing water with shredded coconut. This mixture is strained through cheesecloth to filter out the coconut pieces.

*Yields 1 serving*
Calories: 307
Fat: 1 gram
Protein: 14 grams
Carbohydrates: 63 grams
Cholesterol: 5 milligrams

1 cup canned unsweetened
    pineapple chunks
1 cup coconut water
½ cup nonfat yogurt
½ cup skim milk

# 5

# Breads

# Low-Calorie Corn Bread

The cream-style corn and cheddar cheese make this corn bread so decadent you won't believe it's so low in calories.

**Yields 10 servings**
Calories: 151
Fat: 6 grams
Protein: 5 grams
Carbohydrates: 20 grams
Cholesterol: 36 milligrams

1 cup self-rising yellow cornmeal mix
2 tablespoons sugar
4 tablespoons butter, melted and divided
¾ cup fat-free sour cream
1 cup no-salt-added cream-style corn
½ cup shredded reduced-fat extra-sharp
    cheddar cheese
1 whole egg
2 egg whites
light cooking spray

1. Preheat oven to 425°F.

2. Combine cornmeal mix and sugar in a large bowl.

3. Combine butter, sour cream, creamed corn, cheese, egg, and egg whites in a medium bowl. Stir well with a whisk. Add to cornmeal mixture, stirring until moist.

4. Pour batter into a 13" x 9" baking pan coated with cooking spray.

5. Bake for 25 minutes.

# Oatmeal Banana Bread

You can replace the soy milk with yogurt if you prefer.

**Yields 20 servings**
Calories: 117
Fat: 4 grams
Protein: 3 grams
Carbohydrates: 19 grams
Cholesterol: 21 milligrams

light cooking spray
1½ cups flour
⅔ cup sugar
1½ teaspoons baking powder
¼ teaspoon baking soda
¼ teaspoon salt
¾ cup dry oatmeal
1 cup mashed bananas
½ cup soy milk
¼ cup walnut oil
1 teaspoon vanilla extract
2 eggs

1. Preheat oven to 350°F.

2. Spray an 8" x 4" loaf pan with the light cooking spray.

3. Mix all dry ingredients in a large bowl.

4. Mix the mashed banana, soy milk, oil, vanilla, and eggs in a small bowl.

5. Blend the wet ingredients in with the dry ingredients.

6. Spoon batter into the prepared pan and bake for 50 minutes or until light golden brown on top.

7. Cool on a wire rack for 20 minutes.

8. Remove the bread from the pan and cool thoroughly on the rack before serving.

# Irish Soda Bread

This is a low-calorie version of traditional Irish soda bread, using fat-free milk instead of buttermilk.

1. Mix the dry ingredients in a medium bowl.

2. Mix the wet ingredients in a medium bowl.

3. Add the wet ingredients to the dry ingredients and mix until batter forms a doughy consistency.

4. Knead the dough on a lightly floured surface for approximately 4 minutes. Form into an 8" round.

5. Cut the round into quarters.

6. Place each quarter on a lightly oiled frying pan.

7. Fry on medium heat, cooking each side about 4 minutes.

*Yields 8 servings*
Calories: 67
Fat: <1 gram
Protein: 3 grams
Carbohydrates: 13 grams
Cholesterol: <1 milligram

*1 cup self-rising flour*
*½ teaspoon salt*
*1 teaspoon baking soda*
*1 tablespoon lemon juice*
*1 cup fat-free milk*

# Zucchini Loaf

You can replace the honey with Splenda and add more
Splenda if the batter doesn't seem sweet enough.

1. Preheat oven to 350°F.

2. Spray two bread pans with light cooking spray and lightly flour them.

3. Combine flour, baking powder, baking soda, salt, cinnamon, and nutmeg in a medium bowl.

4. Combine milk, egg whites, applesauce, honey, and zucchini in a separate large bowl.

5. Gradually mix the wet ingredients and the dry ingredients.

6. Pour batter into the pans and bake for 1 hour.

*Yields 18 servings*
Calories: 119
Fat: <1 gram
Protein: 3 grams
Carbohydrates: 27 grams
Cholesterol: <1 milligram

*light cooking spray*
*3 cups flour*
*1 tablespoon baking powder*
*½ teaspoon baking soda*
*1½ teaspoons salt*
*2½ teaspoons cinnamon*
*2 teaspoons nutmeg*
*½ cup fat-free milk*
*2 teaspoons whipped egg whites*
*½ cup applesauce*
*½ cup honey*
*2½ cups grated zucchini*

# Orange Cracked-Wheat Bread

*Orange juice adds a nice tang to this bread and helps offset the strong flavor some whole wheat breads can have.*

**Yields 20 servings**
Calories: 87
Fat: 2 grams
Protein: 2 grams
Carbohydrates: 16 grams
Cholesterol: 4 milligrams

½ cup cracked wheat
1 cup boiling water
¼ cup butter
3 tablespoons honey
½ cup orange juice
1 teaspoon grated orange zest
½ teaspoon salt
1 cup whole wheat flour
1.25-ounce package instant dry yeast
2½ to 3½ cups bread flour

1. Pour cracked wheat into large bowl. Pour boiling water over, stir, and let stand for 20 minutes. Add butter and stir until melted. Add honey, orange juice, orange zest, and salt and mix well. Stir in whole wheat flour and instant dry yeast and beat for 2 minutes. Gradually stir in enough bread flour to make a medium-soft dough.

2. Turn dough onto floured surface and knead for 5 to 8 minutes or until elastic. Place in greased bowl, turning to grease top. Cover and let rise in warm place for 1 hour. Punch down dough, divide into two parts, cover with bowl, and let stand for 10 minutes.

3. Grease two 9" × 5" loaf pans with unsalted butter. On lightly floured surface, roll or pat dough to 7" × 12" rectangles. Roll up tightly, starting with 7" side; pinch ends and edges to seal. Place in prepared pans, cover, and let rise until bread fills pans, about 35 minutes.

4. Preheat oven to 350°F. Bake bread for 35 to 45 minutes, or until deep golden brown. Turn out onto wire racks to cool completely.

### Regular Yeast or Instant?

If a recipe calls for dissolving the yeast in a small amount of warm water before adding to the remaining ingredients, you can use regular yeast or cake yeast. If the yeast is added to the ingredients along with the all-purpose flour, be sure to use instant yeast; it dissolves more easily in the smaller amount of liquid available in a batter.

# Olive Loaf Bread

*You can toast this bread and serve it with soup for dipping—delish! This is also a superb bread to give as a gift. Wrap a loaf in a tea towel, using the ends to tie it up.*

1. Mix the coarse-ground wheat, whole wheat flour, yeast, and water in a large bowl. Cover and let rise for 5 hours.

2. Mix the honey, olive oil, and salt with the risen dough.

3. Add the white flour ½ cup at a time until the dough is so thick you can no longer stir it.

4. Knead the remaining flour into the dough inside the bowl.

5. Chop the olives, then mix with the garlic and black pepper in a small bowl.

6. Knead the olive mixture into the dough.

7. Cover dough again and let rise for another 2 hours.

8. Sprinkle a little white flour on a clean work surface and place risen dough on top.

9. Separate the dough into five equal loaves and space evenly on baking sheets. Let the loaves rise another 2 hours.

10. Bake loaves for 30–40 minutes.

*Yields 50 servings*
Calories: 168
Fat: 3 grams
Protein: 5 grams
Carbohydrates: 32 grams
Cholesterol: 0 milligrams

*3 cups dry cracked wheat grain*
*5½ cups fresh whole wheat flour*
*5 teaspoons instant yeast*
*6¼ cups water*
*½ cup honey*
*⅓ cup olive oil*
*5 teaspoons salt*
*7 cups white bread flour*
*30 olives, pitted*
*2 tablespoons chopped garlic*
*1 teaspoon freshly ground black pepper*

# Oatmeal Cinnamon Raisin Bread

*Once baked, you can brush each loaf again with butter
and sprinkle with more cinnamon and sugar to taste.*

**Yields 30 servings**
Calories: 137
Fat: 2 grams
Protein: 3 grams
Carbohydrates: 27 grams
Cholesterol: 17 milligrams

1½ cups dry oats
1½ cups boiling water
4 tablespoons honey
1 tablespoon Splenda brown sugar
   blend
2 teaspoons salt
1 tablespoon instant yeast
2 eggs
½ cup raisins
4 cups unbleached white flour
3 tablespoons melted butter
1 cup Splenda sugar blend
2 tablespoons cinnamon

1. Cook oats in boiling water.

2. Turn the heat off and add the honey, Splenda brown sugar, and salt to the oatmeal while it's still hot.

3. Let cool, then pour the mixture into a large bowl and add the yeast, eggs, raisins, and flour.

4. Once mixture reaches a dough consistency, knead for 10 minutes.

5. Cover bowl and let it rise until dough doubles in size.

6. Remove dough from bowl and cut in half.

7. Mold each half into a rectangle, brush with melted butter, and sprinkle with the cinnamon and sugar mixture.

8. Tuck loaves in two lightly greased loaf pans. Allow loaves to rise until double in size.

9. Preheat oven to 375°F, then bake for 35 minutes.

10. Remove from pan and cool on racks. Brush with additional melted butter.

# Three-Grain Sourdough Bread

*The sour cream, orange juice, and vinegar add a sour flavor to this hearty bread. Be sure to use bread flour for best results.*

1. In large bowl, combine yeast, warm water, and sugar and let stand for 10 minutes. Add salt, sour cream, orange juice, vinegar, oat bran, wheat flour, and rye flour and beat for 2 minutes. Stir in enough bread flour to make a firm dough.

2. On floured surface, knead dough until smooth and elastic, about 8 to 10 minutes. Place dough in greased bowl, turning to grease top of the dough. Cover and let rise for 1 hour, until doubled.

3. Grease two 9" x 5" loaf pans with unsalted butter and set aside. Punch down dough and divide into two pieces; let stand for 10 minutes. Roll or pat dough to 7" x 12" rectangles and roll up tightly, starting with 7" side. Pinch edges to seal; place in prepared pans. Cover and let rise for 30 to 40 minutes, until doubled.

4. Preheat oven to 375°F. Bake bread for 30 to 40 minutes or until loaves are deep golden brown and sound hollow when tapped with fingers. Turn out onto wire rack and brush with more melted butter. Cool completely.

## Why Bread Flour?

When a bread recipe calls for ingredients like whole-grain flours, whole grains like cracked wheat, or rolled oats, using bread flour will make a better bread. These extra ingredients "cut" the gluten as it forms, making a weaker structure. Bread flour contains more gluten so it will compensate for this effect, making nicely grained loaves that slice well.

**_Yields 32 servings_**
Calories: 90
Fat: 3 grams
Protein: 3 grams
Carbohydrates: 15 grams
Cholesterol: 5 milligrams

*2 0.25-ounce packages dry yeast*
*1½ cups warm water*
*1 tablespoon sugar*
*2 teaspoons salt*
*1 cup sour cream*
*1 tablespoon orange juice*
*2 tablespoons apple-cider vinegar*
*⅓ cup oat bran*
*1 cup whole wheat flour*
*1 cup rye flour*
*2 to 3 cups bread flour*
*2 tablespoons butter, melted*

# 6

# Muffins

# Apple-Cinnamon Muffins

*Yields 6 servings*
Calories: 255
Fat: 3 grams
Protein: 8 grams
Carbohydrates: 64 grams
Cholesterol: 2 milligrams

*2 cups dry oat bran*
*¼ cup brown sugar*
*1 tablespoon baking powder*
*2 egg whites*
*1 cup buttermilk*
*½ cup molasses*
*½ cup unsweetened applesauce*
*1 cup chopped apple*
*4 tablespoons cinnamon*

*If you like more cinnamon flavor, fold the apple chunks in 4 tablespoons of cinnamon powder in addition to the cinnamon you sprinkle on top of the muffins before you bake them.*

1. Preheat oven to 450°F.

2. Mix the oat bran, brown sugar, and baking powder in a large bowl.

3. Beat egg whites in a small bowl until foamy. Stir in buttermilk and molasses.

4. Add the buttermilk mixture to the oat bran mixture, then fold in the applesauce and chopped apple.

5. Pour an equal amount of batter into each cup and sprinkle with cinnamon. Bake until tops are golden, about 20 minutes.

# Cherry-Berry Scones

*Yields 8 servings*
Calories: 248
Fat: 8 grams
Protein: 8 grams
Carbohydrates: 36 grams
Cholesterol: 69 milligrams

*2½ cups all-purpose flour*
*2½ teaspoons baking powder*
*1 tablespoon sugar*
*1 teaspoon salt*
*4 tablespoons unsalted butter*
*2 whole eggs, beaten*
*⅔ cup skim milk*
*½ cup frozen cherries, thawed*
*½ cup frozen blueberries, thawed*
*4 egg whites*

*Make these in a skillet for a slightly crunchier texture. It's a quicker way to make them if you need to save some time.*

1. Preheat oven to 450°F.

2. Combine flour, baking powder, sugar, and salt in a large bowl. Cut the butter into small bits and mix with the flour until mixture is crumbly.

3. Add whole eggs, milk, and fruit and mix until blended well.

4. Sprinkle flour over a clean, flat work space and knead the dough into an 8" circle. Cut the circle into eight wedges and transfer to a nonstick baking sheet. Brush top of scone wedges with the egg whites.

5. Bake 15–20 minutes or until scones turn golden.

### Serving Scones
Scones are traditionally served with preserves and clotted cream, but serve these delicious scones with jam or honey to save on calories. They are popular teatime snacks, but they also work well for breakfast.

# Blueberry Muffins

*Sprinkle some powdered sugar on these muffins to make them pop in your mouth.*

1. Preheat oven to 400°F. Prepare a muffin tin with light cooking spray.

2. Mix the flour, sugar, baking powder, baking soda, and salt in a medium bowl.

3. Whisk buttermilk and egg together. Then add the butter and beat well. Add to flour mixture. Fold in the blueberries.

4. Spoon batter into 12 muffin cups and bake for 20 minutes or until the muffins spring back when touched.

## Muffin Tips
A great way to make sure all of your muffins are the exact same size is to use an ice cream scoop to spoon the batter into the tins. For high rising, rounded tops on muffins, preheat your oven to 500°F. As soon as you put the muffins into the oven, decrease the temperature and keep an eye on the muffins because the baking time will go down.

*Yields 12 servings*
Calories: 197
Fat: 8 grams
Protein: 4 grams
Carbohydrates: 27 grams
Cholesterol: 39 milligrams

*light cooking spray*
*2 cups flour*
*½ cup sugar*
*1 teaspoon baking powder*
*½ teaspoon baking soda*
*½ teaspoon salt*
*1 cup low-fat buttermilk*
*1 egg*
*½ cup butter, softened*
*1 cup blueberries*

# Oatmeal Muffins

*If you want to add a little more sweetness, mix some Splenda with cinnamon and sprinkle on top before you bake. The muffins will brown nicely with a crisp sweetness to the tongue.*

1. Preheat oven to 375°F. Line a muffin pan with paper baking cups.

2. Mix flour, oatmeal, Splenda brown sugar blend, baking powder, and salt together in a medium bowl.

3. Combine vanilla extract, skim milk, egg, and applesauce in a small bowl.

4. Add the vanilla, milk, egg, and applesauce mixture to the flour mixture and beat until ingredients are well blended.

5. Pour an equal amount of batter into each cup.

6. Bake 20–25 minutes until lightly browned.

*Yields 12 servings*
Calories: 163
Fat: 2 grams
Protein: 5 grams
Carbohydrates: 30 grams
Cholesterol: 18 milligrams

*2 cups uncooked oatmeal*
*1½ cups flour*
*6 tablespoons Splenda brown sugar blend*
*1 tablespoon baking powder*
*½ teaspoon salt*
*2 tablespoons vanilla extract*
*1 cup skim milk*
*1 egg*
*½ cup unsweetened applesauce*

# Triple-Play Chocolate Banana Nut Muffins

These muffins pack a punch with the crunch of the
nuts and the sweetness of the chocolate and bananas.

*Yields 20 servings*
Calories: 183
Fat: 4 grams
Protein: 5 grams
Carbohydrates: 37 grams
Cholesterol: <1 milligram

*2 cups wheat bran*
*1 cup oat bran*
*1 cup boiling water*
*½ cup applesauce*
*1 cup honey*
*2 egg whites*
*2 cups skim milk*
*2 cups flour*
*3 teaspoons baking soda*
*½ teaspoon salt*
*½ cup chopped walnuts*
*1 cup mashed banana*
*½ cup semi-sweet chocolate chips*

1. Preheat oven to 400°F.

2. Mix boiling water and bran and let stand.

3. Cream applesauce and honey. Add egg whites and milk, then add the bran. Add the flour, soda, and salt. Fold in nuts, mashed bananas, and chocolate chips.

4. Pour an equal amount of batter into each cup. Bake for 20 minutes.

# Raisin Muffins

If you want to dissolve the sugar in the raisins, you can soak them in water for about an hour.

1. Preheat oven to 450°F.

2. Mix the oat bran, brown sugar, and baking powder in a large bowl.

3. Beat egg whites until foamy in a small bowl. Stir in buttermilk and molasses.

4. Add the buttermilk mixture to the oat bran mixture, then fold in the applesauce and raisins.

5. Pour an equal amount of batter into each cup. Bake until tops are golden, about 20 minutes.

## Raisins

There are many different types of raisins. If you like a sweet raisin, the golden raisins are best. If you like a tart or tangy flavor, the black, dark raisins are best. Raisins are dried grapes, but the way they are dried determines the color. Both golden and dark raisins are made from Thompson variety grapes, but the dark raisins are dried in the sun, while golden raisins are oven-dried.

*Yields 6 servings*
Calories: 282
Fat: 3 grams
Protein: 9 grams
Carbohydrates: 71 grams
Cholesterol: 2 milligrams

2 cups dry oat bran
¼ cup brown sugar
1 tablespoon baking powder
2 egg whites
1 cup low-fat buttermilk
½ cup molasses
½ cup unsweetened applesauce
¾ cup raisins

# Cranberry Muffins

This recipe yields very small muffins—or you can simply give each muffin tin
double the batter and make 6 large muffins. If you use double batter
in 6 large muffin tins, bake the muffins for 10 minutes longer.

### Yields 12 servings
Calories: 193
Fat: 1 gram
Protein: 7 grams
Carbohydrates: 38 grams
Cholesterol: <1 milligram

light cooking spray
1½ cups flour
1 cup dry oats
¾ cup sugar
1 teaspoon baking powder
1 teaspoon baking soda
2 tablespoons water
½ cup fat-free milk
2 teaspoons vanilla extract
2 egg whites, lightly beaten
1 cup whole cranberries, fresh or
    frozen

1. Preheat oven to 375°F. Prepare a muffin tin with light cooking spray.

2. Mix flour, oats, sugar, baking powder, and baking soda in a large bowl.

3. Mix the water, milk, vanilla, egg whites, and cranberries in a medium bowl.

4. Add the wet ingredients to the dry ingredients and mix well.

5. Transfer batter to muffin cups. Bake for 20 minutes or until muffin tops are
   lightly browned.

## Smooth Muffins

If you want to add a silky texture without adding fat, you can mix in about ½ cup of pureed
prunes or puree prune baby food. Low-calorie muffins are often drier and coarser than their
full-calorie counterparts because they are missing fat and sugar.

# Oat Bran Muffins

Go nuts! Add ½ cup of walnuts or any type of nut you love.

1. Preheat oven to 400°F. Prepare a muffin tin with light cooking spray.

2. Mix flour, oat bran, Splenda brown sugar, baking powder, and cinnamon in a mixer at low speed.

3. In a small bowl, combine the applesauce, water, oil, and egg whites. Whip these with a fork to blend.

4. Add the wet ingredients to the flour mixture and mix on low or medium speed.

5. Fill muffin tins and bake for 20 minutes or until muffin tops are lightly browned.

## Hot, Hot, Hot!

Serve these muffins still steaming hot from the oven. Cut each down the middle and add a few chocolate chips, then press the halves back together. The melted chocolate will spread into the muffin and add to the sweetness.

**Yields 12 servings**
Calories: 189
Fat: 10 grams
Protein: 11 grams
Carbohydrates: 23 grams
Cholesterol: 0 milligrams

light cooking spray
1 cup flour
1 cup oat bran
½ cup Splenda brown sugar
4 teaspoons baking powder
1 teaspoon ground cinnamon
½ cup unsweetened applesauce
½ cup water
⅓ cup vegetable oil
2 large egg whites

# Pumpkin Muffins

*Add ½ cup of golden raisins if you want a little to chew on in these muffins.*

**Yields 18 servings**
Calories: 124
Fat: 5 grams
Protein: 3 grams
Carbohydrates: 32 grams
Cholesterol: 34 milligrams

*light cooking spray*
*2½ cups flour*
*½ cup Splenda brown sugar*
*1 tablespoon baking powder*
*1 teaspoon ground cinnamon*
*½ teaspoon ground nutmeg*
*½ teaspoon ground ginger*
*¼ teaspoon salt*
*1 cup plain canned pumpkin pie*
*    filling*
*¾ cup fat-free milk*
*2 eggs*
*6 tablespoons butter, melted*

1. Preheat oven to 400°F. Prepare a muffin tin with light cooking spray.

2. Combine flour, Splenda brown sugar, baking powder, cinnamon, nutmeg, ginger, and salt in a large bowl.

3. Stir pumpkin filling, milk, eggs, and melted butter in a medium bowl.

4. Add pumpkin mixture to flour mixture and mix until all ingredients are moistened.

5. Spoon into prepared muffin tin, filling each cup ⅔ full. Bake 15–20 minutes or until muffin tops are golden brown.

# Orange-Pecan Muffins

If you love the taste of orange, add ¼ cup of orange marmalade and/or ¼ cup of grated orange rind.

1. Preheat oven to 400°F. Prepare a muffin tin with light cooking spray.

2. Combine flour, Splenda, baking powder, salt, and baking soda in a large bowl.

3. Beat eggs in a small bowl. Stir yogurt, orange juice, and melted butter in with the eggs.

4. Add the wet ingredients to the dry ingredients, mixing gradually. Fold in pecans.

5. Spoon batter into muffin tins and bake for 20 minutes or until muffin tops are golden.

## Muffins are Welsh

The muffins we know today originated in Wales. They were made with yeast, then set to rise and cooked on a griddle. They date back to the tenth or eleventh century in Wales.

*Yields 12 servings*
Calories: 190
Fat: 10 grams
Protein: 5 grams
Carbohydrates: 20 grams
Cholesterol: 46 milligrams

*light cooking spray*
*2 cups flour*
*⅓ cup Splenda sugar*
*4 teaspoons baking powder*
*½ teaspoon salt*
*¼ teaspoon baking soda*
*2 eggs*
*¾ cup nonfat yogurt*
*¼ cup orange juice*
*¼ cup butter, melted*
*¾ cup chopped pecans*

# Apricot Muffins

**_Yields 12 servings_**
Calories: 296
Fat: 18 grams
Protein: 8 grams
Carbohydrates: 26 grams
Cholesterol: 35 milligrams

_light cooking spray_
_3 tablespoons melted margarine_
_½ cup honey_
_2 eggs, beaten_
_2 bananas, mashed_
_¾ teaspoon baking soda_
_¼ teaspoon salt_
_3 cups almond flour_
_¾ cup chopped almonds_
_½ cup dried apricots_

Almond flour is made with blanched almonds. You can buy it in your local grocery store or make it at home. Simply blend the blanched almonds in a blender or food processor until it's powdery. If you blend further you could have almond butter.

1. Preheat oven to 325°F. Prepare a muffin tin with light cooking spray.

2. Mix margarine, honey, eggs, and bananas in a large bowl. Add baking soda and salt to mixture. Add in almond flour in parts, mixing as you go. Mix in chopped nuts and dried apricots.

3. Spoon batter into the muffin tin. Bake for 30 minutes or until muffins tops are golden brown.

# Raspberry Muffins

**_Yields 12 servings_**
Calories: 13
Fat: <1 gram
Protein: 3 grams
Carbohydrates: 30 grams
Cholesterol: <1 milligram

_light cooking spray_
_2 cups flour_
_1 tablespoon baking powder_
_½ teaspoon salt_
_½ cup sugar_
_¼ cup Egg Beaters_
_½ cup fat-free milk_
_¼ cup pureed prunes_
_1 cup raspberries, frozen or fresh_

Make sure you purchase prunes that have already been pitted before you puree them.

1. Preheat oven to 375°F. Prepare a muffin tin with light cooking spray.

2. Mix the flour, baking powder, salt, and sugar in a medium-sized bowl. Blend in all other ingredients, except the berries, to a lumpy consistency. Add berries to mixture, gently folding in.

3. Spoon muffin batter into the muffin tin and bake 20–30 minutes or until muffin tops are golden brown.

### Raspberries
Raspberries are used to flavor vinegar, wine, champagne, liqueurs, and spirits. They can also be cooked and made into jellies and jams. Raspberries are a summer fruit, and many farms allow visitors to pick fresh berries themselves. Look for bright red berries.

# 7

# Appetizers

# Spinach Puffs

You can add Splenda, sugar, or honey to taste to sweeten the puffs.
You can also substitute crab meat for the spinach to make crab puffs.

**Yields 4 servings**
Calories: 388
Fat: 36 grams
Protein: 9 grams
Carbohydrates: 8 grams
Cholesterol: 23 milligrams

¾ cup chopped mushrooms,
    including stems
¼ cup canola oil
1 5-ounce package frozen chopped
    spinach, thawed, water
    squeezed out
¾ cup shredded Gruyere cheese
2 thawed puff pastry sheets
¼ cup low-cholesterol margarine

1.  Sauté mushrooms in canola oil.

2.  Stir mushrooms with spinach and cheese.

3.  Brush one pastry sheet with margarine.

4.  Spread half spinach mixture on one pastry sheet.

5.  Cover with the remaining pastry sheet.

6.  Top with remaining spinach.

7.  Cover and refrigerate for at least an hour.

8.  Cut into four 1" wheels, like a pizza slice.

9.  Bake on cookie sheet for 15 minutes or until brown.

# White Bean Bruschetta

You can use French bread instead of Italian bread to
make this vegetarian- and vegan-friendly appetizer.

**Yields 6 servings**
Calories: 355
Fat: 6 grams
Protein: 6 grams
Carbohydrates: 25 grams
Cholesterol: 0 milligrams

1 15-ounce can cannelloni beans,
    rinsed and drained
⅓ teaspoon thyme
¼ teaspoon seasoned salt
ground pepper to taste
2 tablespoons chopped Vidalia
    onion
1 small clove garlic, crushed
1 loaf Italian bread, cut into 12 1"
    slices
⅓ cup low-cholesterol margarine,
    melted

1.  Put beans, thyme, salt, pepper, onions, and garlic in a blender or food processor. Puree until smooth.

2.  Lightly spread margarine on bread.

3.  Spread bean paste on each slice of bread.

4.  Place slices of bread under broiler for 1 minute or serve cold.

# Spice and Honey Nuts

*Watch the mixture carefully as it cooks; because it's high in sugar it can burn easily.*

1. Preheat oven to 375°F. Spread walnuts and pecans on large cookie sheet and toast for 8 to 12 minutes or until the nuts are fragrant, stirring once during cooking time.

2. In small saucepan, combine butter, honey, and remaining ingredients over medium heat. Cook, stirring frequently, just until mixture comes to a boil. Drizzle over nuts, tossing to coat. Reduce oven temperature to 325°F. Bake nuts for 15 to 20 minutes, stirring every 5 minutes, until glazed. Cool completely, then break apart and store in airtight container.

## Nut Nutrition

Some nuts may help reduce the risk of heart disease. These include almonds, peanuts, pecans, pistachio nuts, walnuts, and hazelnuts. They are a high-fat food, but the type of fat is mono-unsaturated, which can help lower LDL cholesterol (the "bad" cholesterol).

*Yields 16 servings*
Calories: 220
Fat: 19 grams
Protein: 3 grams
Carbohydrates: 12 grams
Cholesterol: 6 milligrams

*2 cups walnut halves*
*2 cups pecan halves*
*3 tablespoons butter*
*¼ cup honey*
*⅓ cup brown sugar*
*1 teaspoon cinnamon*
*1 teaspoon ginger*
*½ teaspoon cardamom*
*⅛ teaspoon cayenne pepper*

# Honey and Cheese-Stuffed Figs

*You can also marinate the figs in ½ cup of your favorite cognac or other alcohol.*

1. Preheat oven to 300°F.

2. Wash and dry figs. Make a slit in each one from top to bottom.

3. Stuff each fig with the cheese.

4. Roll each fig in olive oil and shake excess off.

5. Bake figs, watching them until they plump up, about 30 minutes.

6. Drizzle honey on baked figs when ready to serve.

*Yields 4 servings*
Calories: 183
Fat: 4 grams
Protein: 3 grams
Carbohydrates: 37 grams
Cholesterol: 9 milligrams

*8 medium ripe figs*
*⅓ cup crumbled Gorgonzola cheese*
*1 teaspoon olive oil*
*¼ cup honey*

# Tomato Bruschetta

Bruschetta is a great appetizer during the fresh tomato season.
It's easy to prepare and bursts with flavor.

*Yields 4 servings*
Calories: 163
Fat: 8 grams
Protein: 4 grams
Carbohydrates: 20 grams
Cholesterol: 0 milligrams

1 14.5-ounce can diced tomatoes
2 scallions, chopped
2 tablespoons olive oil
ground pepper and kosher salt to
taste
½ teaspoon crushed fresh basil
leaves
1 loaf Italian bread, cut into 1"
slices
1 spritz canola oil spray

1.  Mix tomatoes, chopped onions, olive oil, salt, pepper, and basil leaves.

2.  Spread mixture on eight 1" slices of bread lightly covered with canola oil spray.

3.  Broil bread until brown and serve.

### Preparing Tomatoes
Core your tomato before cutting or dicing. Then season them with freshly ground black pepper and let them soak in the pepper for about 20 minutes. This gives the tomato the most pungent summer taste.

# Grilled Vegetable Focaccia

The Focaccia bread can be heated under a broiler for 1 minute, but it's just as good served cold.

*Yields 4 servings*
Calories: 425
Fat: 24 grams
Protein: 8 grams
Carbohydrates: 44 grams
Cholesterol: 0 milligrams

4 pieces sourdough focaccia bread
¼ pound marinated kalamata
olives
½ cup marinated Sicilian cracked
green olives
½ cup roasted red peppers
1 7-ounce can diced tomatoes
2 tablespoons olive oil
kosher salt and ground pepper to
taste
½ teaspoon Italian seasoning

1.  Mix all ingredients except bread together in a large bowl.

2.  Spread mixture on Focaccia bread.

# Cheese Straws

Have fun with these! You can cut them thick or thin and twist
them tightly or loosely before you place on baking sheet.

1. Preheat oven to 350°F.

2. Prepare piecrust mix according to directions.

3. Sprinkle shredded cheese over piecrust dough, then work it into the dough with your hands.

4. Roll dough into a circle, about 8" around, ⅓" thick.

5. Cut long strips about 1" wide.

6. Sprinkle both sides of each strip with cayenne pepper.

7. Place strips on baking sheet, lightly sprayed with cooking spray.

8. Bake until slightly brown.

*Yields 6 servings*
Calories: 350
Fat: 23 grams
Protein: 6 grams
Carbohydrates: 30 grams
Cholesterol: 2 milligrams

*1 15-ounce package piecrust mix*
*½ cup shredded low-fat cheddar*
*cheese*
*½ teaspoon cayenne pepper*
*light cooking spray*

# Deviled Eggs with Capers

If deviled eggs aren't spicy, they aren't devilish enough! This recipe can be adapted if you want less
heat. Deviled eggs are easy to make and transportable—great for a picnic or brunch!

1. Scoop out egg yolks and place in a food processor along with mayonnaise, seasonings, pepper, and capers. Blend until smooth and spoon into the hollows in the eggs.

2. Add the garnish of paprika or chives and chill, covered with aluminum foil tented above the egg yolk mixture.

### Brine-Packed Capers
Capers are actually berries that have been pickled. You can get them packed in salt, but they
are better when packed in brine. You can get larger ones or very, very small ones—the tiny
ones are tastier.

*Yields 12 servings*
Calories: 69
Fat: 6 grams
Protein: 3 grams
Carbohydrates: 0 milligrams

*6 hard-boiled eggs, shelled and*
*halved*
*½ cup low-fat mayonnaise*
*1 teaspoon red hot pepper sauce*
*1 teaspoon celery salt*
*1 teaspoon onion powder*
*1 teaspoon garlic powder*
*1 chili pepper, finely minced, or to*
*taste*
*2 tablespoons capers, extra small*
*garnish of paprika or chopped*
*chives*

# Grilled Herbed Tomatoes

This is a super-fast, super-yummy snack or appetizer and is especially great during the summer months when you want something light and quick.

*Yields 4 servings*
Calories: 56
Fat: 2 grams
Protein: 2 grams
Carbohydrates: 11 grams
Cholesterol: 0 milligrams

*4 large tomatoes*
*2 teaspoons Italian seasoning*
*1 teaspoon olive oil*
*2 teaspoons minced garlic*
*⅓ cup balsamic vinegar*
*coarse salt and pepper to taste*

1. Cut tomatoes into slices ½" thick.

2. Mix Italian seasoning, olive oil, garlic, and vinegar in large bowl.

3. Marinate tomatoes in mixture for at least 1 hour.

4. Preheat the broiler. Arrange tomato slices on baking sheet and place under broiler. Broil until tops are slightly crisp or warmed through. Flip over and broil underside of tomatoes.

### Fruit or Vegetable

The tomato is traditionally thought of as a vegetable, but in fact it is a fruit. Tomatoes are indigenous to the Americas and were not introduced to Europe until the sixteenth century. The British feared the fruit might be poisonous and it did not become popular there until the mid-eighteenth century.

# Super-Skinny Stuffed Mushrooms

Soak your mushrooms in an alcohol of your choice, like red or white wine, for about 1 hour and your taste buds will dance.

*Serves 4–6*
Calories: 202
Fat: 10 grams
Protein: 19 grams
Carbohydrates: 13 grams
Cholesterol: 46 milligrams

*1 16-ounce package reduced-fat*
    *pork sausage*
*½ onion, minced*
*½ minced green pepper*
*1 8-ounce package reduced-fat*
    *cream cheese*
*juice of 1 lemon*
*20–25 whole mushrooms, stems*
    *removed*

1. Preheat oven to 300°F.

2. Brown sausage thoroughly in a large skillet.

3. Add onion and pepper. Cook, remove from heat, and drain fat.

4. Mix cream cheese with lemon juice and cooled sausage mixture.

5. Stuff each mushroom with mixture.

6. Place on baking sheet and bake for 20 minutes or until mushrooms are soft.

# Mary's Marvelous Marinated Mushrooms

*Replace the vinegar with red wine vinegar or another type
of flavored vinegar to pass on a different flavor.*

1. Place mushroom caps in a sauce pan, cover them with water, and add the lemon juice.

2. Bring to boil. Reduce heat and simmer for 5 minutes.

3. Drain and rinse the mushrooms under cold water and set aside in a bowl.

4. Mix vinegar, olive oil, garlic, bay leaf, and parsley flakes in a saucepan and boil for five about minutes. Add salt and pepper to taste. Pour the vinegar mixture over the mushrooms. Let marinate in the fridge and serve cool.

*Yields 6 servings*
Calories: 84
Fat: 7 grams
Protein: 2 grams
Carbohydrates: 5 grams
Cholesterol: 0 milligrams

*20 small mushroom caps, cleaned
juice from 1 lemon
¾ cup vinegar
3 tablespoons olive oil
1 tablespoon minced garlic
⅓ teaspoon crushed bay leaf
1 teaspoon parsley flakes
salt and pepper to taste*

# Cheese, Olive, and Cherry Tomato Kabobs

*This recipe is tricky. You want to rotate the skewers gently on the
grill and remove them immediately once the cheese starts to melt.*

1. Spray each skewer with the light cooking spray

2. Arrange 1 tomato, 1 olive, and 1 cheese cube on each skewer.

3. Grill skewers for just a few moments until cheese starts to melt, then turn to grill all sides.

*Yields 4 servings*
Calories: 232
Fat: 19 grams
Protein: 14 grams
Carbohydrates: 2 grams
Cholesterol: 51 milligrams

*light cooking spray
6 bamboo skewers soaked in water
6 cherry tomatoes
½ pound jack cheese, cut into 1"
    cubes
6 large green marinated olives*

# Beet and Anchovy Canapé

*Yields 6 servings*
Fat: 1 gram
Protein: 5 grams
Carbohydrates: 24 grams
Cholesterol: 4 milligrams

*1 14.5-ounce can unsalted diced baby beets*
*1 teaspoon onion, minced*
*4 tablespoons lemon juice*
*2 tablespoons chopped anchovies*
*1 5-ounce package Old London Melba Toasts*

These are lovely served on a bed of lettuce with diced tomato to garnish and add color.

1. Mix the baby beets, onion, lemon juice, and anchovies in a small bowl.

2. Spread beet and anchovy mixture on Melba Toasts and serve.

### Anchovy Information
Anchovies are often confused with sardines, but anchovies are smaller. Their scales are virtually nonexistent and also perfectly edible. They are used in many Mediterranean dishes, where they are plentiful. They are related to the herring, and both kinds of fish were traditionally salted for preservation.

# Crunchy Party Mix

*Yields 10 servings*
Calories: 247
Fat: 17 grams
Protein: 6 grams
Carbohydrates: 20 grams
Cholesterol: 0 milligrams

*2 tablespoons peanut oil*
*1 tablespoon minced garlic*
*1 cup unsalted walnuts*
*1 cup unsalted almonds*
*½ cup unsalted pretzel sticks, broken into small pieces*
*1 teaspoon chili powder*
*1½ tablespoons low-sodium soy sauce*
*1 teaspoon cayenne pepper*
*2 teaspoons Splenda*
*sea salt to taste*
*½ cup seedless raisins*

The cayenne pepper adds a spicy kick, but if you prefer your snacks mild you can leave it out.

1. Warm peanut oil and garlic in a heavy skillet.

2. Add all other ingredients except raisins, stirring constantly.

3. When thoroughly warmed and mixed, stir in raisins.

4. Remove from heat. Put into a serving bowl.

5. Chill and serve.

### Healthy Nuts
Buy nuts in small quantities, because they can become rancid fairly quickly. You can store nuts in the freezer, but be sure to thaw them completely before chopping or they will become oily.

# Walnut Cheese Bites

*If you don't love gorgonzola, replace with bleu cheese or even feta. You also might like to use a mixture of each.*

1. Preheat oven to 350°F.

2. Sandwich 1 teaspoon cheese between 2 walnut halves. Place walnuts on a baking sheet.

3. Toast in the oven until cheese starts to melt, about ten minutes.

4. Drizzle honey over walnuts and serve.

## Walnut Preparation

The walnuts in this recipe can be prepared as is, but are best if they are blanched. Boil them in water for about 1 minute and they will be softer and lighter in color. This mellows the walnuts' flavor.

*Yields 4 servings*
Calories: 122
Fat: 10 grams
Protein: 5 grams
Carbohydrates: 6 grams
Cholesterol: 13 milligrams

*12 walnut halves*
*4 ounces gorgonzola cheese*
*1 tablespoon honey to drizzle*

# Chicken "Wings"

*This spicy and savory sauce is perfect with tender chicken. Serve this appetizer with toothpicks for easy dipping.*

1. Cut chicken tenders in half crosswise. In heavy-duty food-storage bag, combine remaining ingredients except sour cream and celery; mix well. Add chicken tenders and seal bag. Place bag in baking dish; refrigerate for at least 8 hours, up to 24 hours.

2. When ready to prepare, preheat oven to 400°F. Drain chicken tenders, reserving marinade. Arrange tenders in single layer in large pan. Drizzle with ½ cup of the reserved marinade. Bake for 20 to 25 minutes or until chicken is thoroughly cooked.

3. Meanwhile, place remaining marinade in small saucepan. Bring to a simmer over high heat, then reduce heat to low and cook for 10 to 15 minutes, stirring frequently, until mixture is syrupy. Combine with sour cream and serve as a dipping sauce for chicken along with celery.

*Yields 10 servings*
Calories: 199
Fat: 4 grams
Protein: 21
Carbohydrates: 17 grams
Cholesterol: 62 milligrams

*2 pounds chicken tenders*
*⅓ cup soy sauce*
*¼ cup apple-cider vinegar*
*2 tablespoons Dijon mustard*
*¼ cup honey*
*¼ cup brown sugar*
*1 teaspoon salt*
*1 teaspoon hot sauce*
*4 cloves garlic, minced*
*½ cup minced onion*
*1 cup low-fat sour cream*
*2 cups celery sticks*

# Rye Boat with Bread Cubes

This is not an especially low-fat recipe, but cheese is high in protein and helps curb your appetite.

*Yields 6 servings*
Calories: 223
Fat: 10 grams
Protein: 12 grams
Carbohydrates: 16 grams
Cholesterol: 30 milligrams

*1 round loaf rye bread*
*1 14-ounce package fondue*
*fondue pot and forks*

1. Cut hole on top of bread and scoop out the bread. Cut the insides into 1" cubes and place them back in the loaf.

2. Prepare fondue according to package directions

3. When fondue is ready, dip the cubes in and eat.

## How to Fondue

Fondue was a classic peasant dish, born in Switzerland as a way to use up aging cheese. Today, packaged fondue is easy because you can melt it according to the directions and it's virtually goof-proof. The best part is you can add nearly anything you like to the cheese, like chopped vegetables, nuts, or even cooked meats.

# Stuffed Cucumbers

Make sure your cucumber is fresh and crisp before you prepare this appetizer. Seedless cucumbers are easiest to work with.

*Yields 4 servings*
Calories: 75
Fat: 5 grams
Protein: 4 grams
Carbohydrates: 5 grams
Cholesterol: 14 milligrams

*2 large cucumbers*
*3 ounces low-fat cream cheese*
*1 tablespoon low-fat bleu cheese*
*1 teaspoon dill*
*1 teaspoon parsley*
*1 teaspoon minced onion*

1. Using a vegetable peeler, create stripes in the cucumber by peeling strips about ¼" apart, lengthwise. Cut ends off each cucumber. Scoop the seeds and pulp out of the cucumber with a melon baller.

2. Mix the cream cheese, blue cheese, dill, parsley, and minced onion in a small bowl.

3. Place mixture inside the hollowed cucumbers using a pastry bag with a star tip.

4. Cover cucumbers with plastic wrap and refrigerate at least 1 hour.

5. Cut cucumbers into 1" circles and serve.

# Light and Little Pizzas

*You can make your own marinara sauce by blending canned or crushed tomatoes with garlic, olive oil, fresh basil, and oregano. Enhance it with onion, carrots, white wine, parsley, and bay leaves added to taste.*

1. Preheat oven to 400°F.

2. Cut a 3" circle in each slice of bread with cookie cutter or drinking glass.

3. Brush bread circles with olive oil and bake until brown, about 6 minutes.

4. Mix marinara sauce and 1 tablespoon Parmesan cheese and spread on bread rounds. Top each with mozzarella cheese. Add a sprinkle of oregano and Parmesan.

5. Bake about 4 minutes or until cheese melts.

## Pizza Stats

Pizza was created in Naples around the third century B.C. Ancient scholars recorded its origins as a flat round of dough dressed with olive oil, herbs, and honey. Other writings describe a sheet of flour filled with cheese and honey, flavored with bay leaves.

*Yields 4 servings*
Calories: 106
Fat: 4 grams
Protein: 7 grams
Carbohydrates: 12 grams
Cholesterol: 13 milligrams

*4 pieces low-carb white bread*
*olive oil to taste*
*⅓ cup low-sodium marinara sauce*
*2 tablespoons grated Parmesan cheese*
*4 ounces grated mozzarella cheese*
*½ teaspoon crushed dried oregano*

# Chicken and Pineapple Finger Sandwiches

Yields 4 servings
Calories: 273
Fat: 10 grams
Protein: 14 grams
Carbohydrates: 34 grams
Cholesterol: 23 milligrams

1 skinless chicken breast
¼ cup nonfat plain yogurt
¼ cup low-fat mayonnaise
1 tablespoon lime juice
1 teaspoon curry powder
4 teaspoons flat-leaf parsley,
    chopped
3 tablespoons sliced almonds
1¼ cup diced pineapple
½ cup watercress without stems
8 pieces thin white or wheat bread

*If you boil a chicken breast that still has a bone in it the chicken will be juicier. Simply remove the bone after boiling.*

1. Cook chicken breast in boiling water about five minutes or until done.

2. While chicken is cooling, mix yogurt, mayonnaise, lime juice, curry powder, parsley, and almonds together.

3. Cut the chicken into bite-sized pieces, then add chicken pieces and pineapple to the mixture.

4. Spread the mixture over slices of bread and sprinkle with watercress to serve sandwiches.

# Cousin Sandy's Cheddar Cheese and Paprika Finger Sandwiches

Yields 2 servings
Calories: 160
Fat: 4 grams
Protein: 10 grams
Carbohydrates: 22 grams
Cholesterol: 5 milligrams

4 ounces shredded low-fat cheddar
    cheese
4 teaspoons Hungarian paprika
1 teaspoon Worcestershire sauce
⅓ teaspoon cayenne pepper
4 pieces thin white bread

*Traditional finger sandwiches are crustless, so cut the crusts off the bread before preparation.*

1. Melt the cheese in the microwave.

2. Mix the paprika, Worcestershire sauce, and cayenne pepper, then fold in with the cheddar cheese.

3. Spread the cheese mixture on the bread and top with the second piece of bread.

# 8

## Dips

# Seven-Layer Mexican Dip

No one will notice that this crowd-pleasing dip has been lightened.
Serve it with baked chips or veggies.

*Yields 12 servings; serving size 2
ounces*
Calories: 78
Fat: 4 grams
Protein: 3 grams
Carbohydrates: 8 grams
Cholesterol: 8 milligrams

*1 cup low-fat sour cream*
*1 tablespoon reduced-sodium taco
    seasoning*
*9 ounces fat-free bean dip*
*¾ cup guacamole*
*½ cup low-fat shredded cheddar
    cheese*
*5 scallions, chopped*
*1 tomato, chopped*
*10 black olives, sliced*

1. Combine the sour cream and taco seasoning.

2. Spread bean dip on the bottom of a round serving bowl or edged platter.

3. Layer the guacamole next, spreading evenly over the bean dip. Layer the sour cream, also spreading evenly.

4. Sprinkle the shredded cheese evenly over the guacamole and top with the scallions, tomatoes, and olives.

# Marinara Dip

This dip is wonderful because it is also very versatile. It can be used as a dip or
even as a sauce to garnish pasta, steamed vegetables, steak, or pork chops.

*Yields 4 servings*
Calories: 35
Fat: 2 grams
Protein: 1 gram
Carbohydrates: 4 grams
Cholesterol: 1 milligrams

*1 8-ounce can diced tomatoes*
*2 cloves garlic, crushed*
*1 teaspoon red pepper flakes*
*1 tablespoon parsley flakes*
*¼ teaspoon lemon juice*
*½ tablespoon anchovy paste*
*½ tablespoon extra virgin olive oil*

1. Heat all ingredients in saucepan and cook over low heat for about 5 minutes or until well blended.

2. Add salt and pepper to taste.

3. Remove from heat, place in a bowl, and serve with baked chips or vegetables.

### Marinara Sauce
Marinara sauce originated in Naples as a meatless sauce used on sailing ships. The lack of meat, sheer simplicity, and high acid content of this sauce means that it does not easily spoil and therefore will keep in the refrigerator for weeks.

# Chunky Vegetable Dip

You can substitute onion soup mix for the vegetable.

1. Boil the carrot, celery, and onion for 2–3 minutes.

2. Remove, drain, and cool vegetables. Chop finely.

3. Mix sour cream with vegetable soup mix and add chopped vegetables.

4. Refrigerate dip for at least 1 hour and serve with chips.

*Yields 4 servings*
Calories: 70
Fat: 0 grams
Protein: 3 grams
Carbohydrates: 16 grams
Cholesterol: 5 milligrams

*1 large carrot*
*2 stalks celery*
*½ Vidalia onion*
*1 8-ounce carton fat-free sour cream*
*1 envelope vegetable soup mix*
*1 bag baked chips*

# Sweet Onion Dip

You can replace the sour cream with fat-free yogurt for a sweeter taste or make a mixture that's half yogurt and half sour cream.

1. Mix all ingredients.

2. Refrigerate for at least one hour.

3. Serve with celery or carrot sticks.

*Yields 4 servings*
Calories: 88
Fat: <1 gram
Protein: 3 grams
Carbohydrates: 20 grams
Cholesterol: 5 milligrams

*1 envelope dry onion mix*
*¼ cup Splenda*
*1 8-ounce carton fat-free sour cream*
*1 teaspoon sweet pickle relish*

## Ravishing Relish

The two most commonly available relish types are hamburger relish, made with a ketchup base, and hotdog relish, made with a mustard base. Gentleman's Relish was invented in 1828 by an Englishman named John Osborn. It contains spiced anchovy, butter, herbs, and spices.

# Yogurt Cheese Spinach Dip

*Yogurt cheese is an excellent substitute for cream cheese in almost any recipe.*
*Be sure you use the simplest yogurt, without gelatin or other thickening agents added.*

*Yields 8 servings*
Calories: 62
Fat: 3 grams
Protein: 4 grams
Carbohydrates: 6 grams
Cholesterol: 4 milligrams

2 cups plain low-fat yogurt
½ cup finely chopped onion
2 cloves garlic, minced
1 tablespoon olive oil
2 cups fresh spinach
½ teaspoon salt
⅛ teaspoon cayenne pepper
2 tablespoons lemon juice

1. The day before you want to serve the dip, place the yogurt in a strainer lined with cheesecloth or a coffee filter. Rest the strainer over a deep bowl, cover both with plastic wrap, and let stand in the refrigerator overnight.

2. The next day, remove the yogurt cheese from the strainer; save the whey for another use.

3. In a heavy saucepan, cook onion and garlic in olive oil over medium heat until tender, about 5 minutes. Coarsely chop the spinach and add to the pan; cook and stir until spinach is wilted and water has evaporated, about 3–4 minutes. Remove from heat and sprinkle with salt, cayenne pepper, and lemon juice. Remove to a medium mixing bowl; let stand until cool, about 45 minutes. Blend in the yogurt cheese. Serve immediately or cover and chill for up to 3 days.

# White Bean Dip

*Toasting the bread in the oven before spreading the bean puree gives this dish a crunchy texture.*

*Yields 4–6 servings*
Calories: 523
Fat: 22 grams
Protein: 13 grams
Carbohydrates: 69 grams
Cholesterol: 0 milligrams

½ cup extra virgin olive oil
2 cloves garlic, crushed
1 French baguette, thinly sliced
1 15-ounce can cannelloni beans or
    garbanzo beans
2 tablespoon crushed rosemary
    leaves
½ teaspoon lemon juice
kosher salt and white pepper to
    taste

1. Mix olive oil and crushed garlic. Spread over bread slices.

2. Combine the remaining ingredients in a food processor and puree.

3. Spread puree over bread.

### Double Duty Dip
This dip can stand alone for dipping vegetables, bread, and crackers, or it can be used as a spread. If you are having guests over, put out bowls of the dip and provide both vegetables and crackers. Place small spreaders on the side and let guests decide how they'd like to enjoy this dip.

# Edamame Dip

Edamame, or soy beans, are rich in protein and highly nutritious. They can also be eaten alone as a snack. Boil them for about 10 minutes, then drain and salt them.

1. Boil edamame in water until tender, adding a little salt as it boils.

2. Meanwhile, mix the garlic, mayonnaise, lemon juice, salt, and pepper. Add the edamame.

3. Puree everything in a food processor or blender until smooth.

4. Serve with fat-free chips or corn chips.

**Yields 4 servings**
Calories: 68
Fat: 4 grams
Protein: 3 grams
Carbohydrates: 6 grams
Cholesterol: 3 milligrams

NOTE: Nutritional information based on the dip without the chips.

1½ cups frozen edamame, thawed
1 crushed clove garlic
¼ cup light mayonnaise
2 tablespoons lemon juice
salt and pepper to taste
1 bag baked chips

# Guacamole Dip

You can use any onion in this recipe, but the Vidalia onion imparts a sweet flavor.

1. Halve the avocados and scoop meat from skins.

2. Mash avocado meat with lime juice.

3. Mix in tomato, jalapeño, garlic, cilantro, and onion.

4. Add salt and pepper to taste.

5. Cover and let stand for 1 hour.

6. Serve with baked tortilla chips.

**Yields 6 servings**
Calories: 181
Fat: 16 grams
Protein: 3 grams
Carbohydrates: 12 grams
Cholesterol: 0 milligrams

3 extra-ripe avocados
juice of 2 limes
½ large tomato, skinned and
    chopped
1 jalapeño pepper, chopped
2 cloves garlic, chopped
3 tablespoons cilantro leaves,
    crushed
1 large Vidalia onion, chopped
salt and pepper to taste

### Guacamole Rico
Guacamole dip dates back to the Aztecs, around the fourteenth century, when avocados, lime juice, and salt were the basic ingredients. Variations today include onions, tomato, garlic, and spices, among others.

# Bread Bowl Dip

You can mix some of the sourdough bread into the dip to add
texture or use the bread to dip along with chopped veggies.

**Yields 4 servings**
Calories: 93
Fat: <1 gram
Protein: 3 grams
Carbohydrates: 21 grams
Cholesterol: 5 milligrams

NOTE: Nutritional information
based on dip without the bread
boule.

1 large sourdough boule
1 8-ounce carton fat-free sour
    cream
1 small Vidalia onion, chopped
1 envelope dry onion soup mix

1. Cut a hole in the top of the bread loaf.

2. Scoop out all the bread in the boule up to ¼" near crust.

3. Refrigerate bread bowl for 1 hour.

4. Mix sour cream, chopped onion, and onion soup mix, then pour the mixture into the cooled bread bowl and serve with baked chips or vegetable strips.

# Gingerbread Fruit Dip

This dip is wonderful served with fresh fruits like apple
and pear slices, banana slices, and strawberries.

**Yields 12 servings**
Calories: 126
Fat: 8 grams
Protein: 2 grams
Carbohydrates: 13 grams
Cholesterol: 26 milligrams

1 8-ounce package cream cheese,
    softened
½ cup low-fat sour cream
⅓ cup brown sugar
¼ cup maple syrup or light
    molasses
2 tablespoons chopped candied
    ginger
½ teaspoon ground ginger
½ teaspoon cinnamon
¼ teaspoon nutmeg

1. In medium bowl, beat cream cheese until light and fluffy. Gradually add sour cream, beating until smooth. Add sugar and beat well. Gradually add molasses and beat until smooth. Stir in remaining ingredients. Cover and chill for at least 3 hours before serving with fresh fruit.

## Candied Ginger
Candied ginger is also known as crystallized ginger. It is made of pieces of ginger root simmered in a sugar syrup, then rolled in sugar. You can make your own by combining ¾ cup sugar with ¾ cup water and bringing to a simmer. Add ½ cup peeled and chopped fresh ginger root; simmer for 25 minutes. Drain, dry, then roll in sugar to coat.

# Dad's Dainty Dill and Cucumber Dip

*This cool, refreshing dip is great on a hot summer day and a superb way to use fresh cucumbers from your garden.*

1. Mix all ingredients together.

2. Refrigerate for several hours.

3. Serve with baked chips.

## Perfect with Proteins

This dip is also a great condiment for broiled salmon, lean flank steak, and grilled chicken. Simply prepare the meat or fish the way you'd like and serve the dip on top or on the side. Save leftovers to use with chips or vegetables.

*Yields 4–6 servings*
Calories: 42
Fat: 1 gram
Protein: 3 grams
Carbohydrates: 6 grams
Cholesterol: <1 milligram

*1 cup plain nonfat yogurt*
*2 large seedless cucumbers, peeled and finely chopped*
*1 tablespoon dill*
*1 teaspoon lemon juice*
*1 teaspoon virgin olive oil*
*salt and pepper to taste*

# Smoked Salmon Dip

*If you like a little kick in your dip, add a few dashes of Tabasco sauce to this recipe.*

1. Mix all ingredients except the salmon until well blended.

2. Chop salmon into small pieces and mix into other ingredients.

3. Add salt and pepper to taste.

4. Refrigerate at least 1 hour, then serve with baked chips or vegetables.

## Healthy Salmon

Salmon is low in calories and saturated fat, yet very high in protein. Salmon is an excellent source of omega-3 fatty acids, which can improve heart function and lower blood pressure. You can get omega-3 fatty acids from most cold-water fish, such as albacore tuna, salmon, and trout, which tend to have more of these good fats than other fish.

*Yields 4 servings*
Calories: 42
Fat: 1 gram
Protein: 3 grams
Carbohydrates: 6 grams
Cholesterol: <1 milligram

*2 small cups fat-free sour cream*
*1 teaspoon lemon juice*
*1½ tablespoons drained capers*
*1 small red onion, finely chopped*
*1 tablespoon tomato paste*
*¼ pound smoked salmon*
*salt and pepper to taste*

# Hot Crab Dip

This meaty and delicious dip is best served with
heated raw vegetables or very light, thin crackers.

1. Mix all ingredients in medium bowl.

2. Heat in microwave for 1 or 2 minutes until hot.

3. Serve with baked chips or vegetables.

*Yields 6 servings*
Calories: 169
Fat: 5 grams
Protein: 14 grams
Carbohydrates: 15 grams
Cholesterol: 46 milligrams

*1 pound crabmeat*
*2 scallions, finely chopped*
*4 ounces fat-free cream cheese,*
*  softened*
*½ cup light mayonnaise*
*¼ cup grated parmesan cheese*
*⅓ teaspoon horseradish*
*salt to taste*

# Broccoli and Cheese Dip

You will love it when guests ask how you make this "cheesy" dip and they discover how easy it is.

1. Melt margarine, cheese, and Worsterchesire sauce in microwave.

2. Boil broccoli until cooked, as directed on package.

3. Mix broccoli and cheese and microwave until hot.

4. Serve with baked chips.

*Yields 6 servings*
Calories: 363
Fat: 31 grams
Protein: 12 grams
Carbohydrates: 11 grams
Cholesterol: 58 milligrams

*1 stick margarine*
*1 16-ounce box reduced-fat*
*  Velveeta jalapeño cheese*
*1 teaspoon Worcestershire sauce*
*1 16-ounce package frozen chopped*
*  broccoli, thawed*

## Creamy and Cheesy

You might be surprised to learn that Velveeta's heritage as cheese is as authentic as its Swiss roots. Swiss immigrant Emil Frey first made Velveeta in 1918 in Monroe, New York, at the Monroe Cheese Company. Later sold to Kraft Foods in 1927, Velveeta is known for its easy melting.

# Cinnamon Curry Fruit Dip

*The sweet tartness of peaches combines beautifully with curry powder.*
*This special dip can be served as dessert.*

1. Peel peach and remove stone; cut peach into slices. Place in food processor or blender along with curry powder, cinnamon, brown sugar, sour cream, and cream cheese and blend until smooth. Place in refrigerator and chill for at least 4 hours before serving. Serve with fruit and bread.

*Yields 8 servings*
Calories: 88
Fat: 6 grams
Protein: 2 grams
Carbohydrates: 9 grams
Cholesterol: 18 milligrams

*1 peach*
*1 teaspoon curry powder*
*½ teaspoon cinnamon*
*¼ cup brown sugar*
*½ cup low-fat sour cream*
*1 3-ounce package cream cheese, softened*

# Artichoke Spinach Dip

*You can add some melted low-fat shredded cheese on top instead of bread crumbs.*

1. Preheat oven to 350°F. Prepare a baking dish with light cooking spray.

2. Sauté the garlic in olive oil.

3. Pulse ricotta cheese, thyme, lemon zest, and cayenne pepper in food processor until creamy.

4. Add artichokes, spinach, and Parmesan cheese; pulse again, but keep it chunky.

5. Transfer artichoke mixture into baking dish sprayed with light cooking spray.

6. Sprinkle bread crumbs and garlic over artichoke mixture. Season with salt and pepper.

7. Bake for 20 minutes or until warmed through.

8. Serve with chips or vegetables.

*Yields 4 servings*
Calories: 225
Fat: 10 grams
Protein: 18 grams
Carbohydrates: 19 grams
Cholesterol: 34 milligrams

*light cooking spray*
*2 cloves garlic, minced*
*1 tablespoon olive oil*
*1½ cups part skim ricotta cheese*
*½ teaspoon thyme*
*1 teaspoon lemon zest*
*½ teaspoon cayenne pepper*
*1 9-ounce box frozen artichokes, thawed and drained*
*8 ounces frozen spinach, thawed and drained*
*¼ cup grated Parmesan cheese*
*¼ cup bread crumbs*
*salt and pepper to taste*

# Black Bean Dip

*This is excellent for parties or as a snack and is also very low in fat.*

**_Yields 8 servings_**
Calories: 36
Fat: 13 grams
Protein: 12 grams
Carbohydrates: 39 grams
Cholesterol: 5 milligrams

*1½ cups black beans, rinsed and
    drained*
*½ cup finely minced Vidalia onion*
*4 cloves garlic, minced*
*2 teaspoons red hot pepper sauce or
    to taste*
*juice of 1 lime*
*½ cup low-fat sour cream*
*½ cup chopped cilantro or parsley*
*salt and pepper to taste*

1. Pulse all ingredients in a food processor or blender. Serve chilled or at room temperature.

# 9

# Soups

# Low-Calorie Vegetable Soup

### Yields 4–6 servings
Calories: 127
Fat: <1 gram
Protein: 6 grams
Carbohydrates: 29 grams
Cholesterol: 0 milligrams

4 cups water
1 pound mixed vegetables, any kind
1 onion, chopped
1 8-ounce can corn
6 celery sticks, chopped
3 tablespoons vegetable bouillon or
   vegetable base
1 28-ounce can crushed tomatoes
4 teaspoons Worcestershire sauce
1 teaspoon black pepper

*Green beans, carrots, broccoli, and cauliflower all make great choices for the mixed vegetables. To make it a meal, add some French bread for dipping.*

1. Bring the water to a boil in a large pot.

2. Add in the mixed vegetables, onion, corn, and celery.

3. Stir in the vegetable bouillon or base.

4. Add the crushed tomatoes, mixing as ingredients boil.

5. Add Worcestershire sauce and black pepper to taste. Let the soup sit and simmer for a while before eating.

# Cabbage Soup

*A lot of people like their cabbage soup spicy. If you like
it this way, add a teaspoon or two of chili pepper.*

1. Bring the broth to a boil in a large pot.

2. Add in the onion and garlic; stir for five minutes, then add the mustard.

3. Stir in cabbage and tomato. Squeeze one lemon into the mixture, continue to stir. Add salt and pepper to taste.

4. Turn heat to simmer for about 10 minutes.

*Yields 4 servings*
Calories: 135
Fat: <1 gram
Protein: 5 grams
Carbohydrates: 28 grams
Cholesterol: 0 milligrams

*5 cups vegetable broth*
*1 onion, thinly sliced*
*3 cloves garlic, crushed*
*1 tablespoon dry mustard*
*1 9-ounce can diced tomatoes*
*1 lemon*
*salt and pepper to taste*
*1 green cabbage, thinly chopped*

# White Bean Soup

*Yields 4 servings*
Calories: 355
Fat: 15 grams
Protein: 17 grams
Carbohydrates: 42 grams
Cholesterol: 0 milligrams

*½ pound dried white beans*
*¼ cup olive oil*
*5 garlic cloves, crushed*
*2 carrots, peeled and chopped*
*2 celery stalks, chopped*
*16 ounces low-sodium chicken broth*
*6 cups water*
*1 bay leaf*
*¼ cup chopped parsley*

*Bean soups can be chunky or pureed. If you prefer a puree, put everything into a blender once it's been cooked, one cup at a time, and blend until creamy.*

1. Cover the beans in a bowl of water and soak overnight in the refrigerator.

2. Drain the beans and place them in a large pot.

3. Add the olive oil, garlic, carrots, celery, chicken broth, and water and bring everything to a boil. Cook for 15 minutes.

4. Reduce heat to a simmer; add the bay leaf and parsley.

5. Continue to simmer until beans are tender, about 2 hours, then serve.

# Chicken Soup

*Chicken soup is truly the simplest recipe in the world. All you need to do is determine how intense you want the broth and add water according to taste if it's too strong.*

1. Heat the olive oil in a large soup pot. Add the onion and sauté until soft.

2. Add the other vegetables and chicken and continue to stir fry for about 10 minutes.

3. Cover with the chicken broth and water and stir everything together.

4. Simmer for 30 minutes and serve.

*Yields 4 servings*
Calories: 190
Fat: 8 grams
Protein: 16 grams
Carbohydrates: 17 grams
Cholesterol: 46 milligrams

*1 tablespoon olive oil*
*1 onion, diced*
*½ pound chicken, diced or chunked raw chicken*
*1 potato, diced*
*4 celery stalks, diced*
*2 carrots, diced*
*16 ounces low-sodium chicken broth*
*4 cups of water*
*salt and pepper to taste*

# Chilled Cucumber and Yogurt Soup

*Make sure to buy seedless cucumbers; they work best with this soup.*

*Yields 6 servings*
Calories: 80
Fat: <1 gram
Protein: 5 grams
Carbohydrates: 15 grams
Cholesterol: 2 milligrams

*4 cups cucumber, peeled and
    chopped*
*2 cups water*
*2 cups nonfat plain yogurt*
*12 fresh mint leaves*
*2 tablespoons honey*
*2 teaspoons salt*
*¼ teaspoon dill weed*
*¼ cup chopped scallions*

1.  Place everything except the scallions in a blender. Blend until the mixture forms a puree.

2.  Serve in bowls and sprinkle with scallions

**Oh, the Possibilities!**
If you're eating on the run, this soup can be made by simply pouring ½ cup fat-free yogurt in a bowl and folding in slices of cucumber. This is a traditionally Turkish soup, to which walnuts and raisins are often added as well.

# Creamy Tomato Soup

*Add the milk slowly to determine how thick or thin you want it. Stop adding it to your own liking.*

1. Combine broth and tomatoes in a blender and puree. Add the heavy cream and half of the milk and puree.

2. Pour the puree into a large, deep skillet and simmer on medium. Add salt and pepper to taste, continue to simmer, stirring occasionally. Add more milk if you want it thinner.

3. Serve in bowls and garnish with parsley.

### Early Tomato Soup

An early version of tomato soup appears in a cookbook compiled by the Ladies' Aid Society of the First Presbyterian Church in Marion, Ohio, in 1894. The recipe calls for six large tomatoes, stewed and passed through a sieve. Butter, cream, flour, cornstarch, scalded milk, salt, pepper, sugar, and mace are added and boiled with the tomatoes to serve.

**Yields 4 servings**
Calories: 150
Fat: 6 grams
Protein: 6 grams
Carbohydrates: 21 grams
Cholesterol: 21 milligrams

16 ounces low-sodium vegetable broth
1 28-ounce can crushed tomatoes
¼ cup heavy cream
1 cup skim milk
salt and pepper to taste
¼ cup fresh chopped parsley

# Curried Butternut Squash

**Yields 8 servings**
Calories: 93
Fat: 5 grams
Protein: 2 grams
Carbohydrates: 12 grams
Cholesterol: 0 milligrams

3 tablespoons margarine
2 onions, sliced
1 tablespoon curry powder
2 butternut squashes, peeled,
    seeded, and cut into small
    chunks
16 ounces low-sodium chicken
    broth
1 teaspoon salt
2 cups water

*This soup can easily be frozen and reheated. Place leftovers in resealable plastic containers. When ready to use, allow to thaw and reheat in a microwave.*

1. Melt the margarine in a large pot. Add the onions and cook for 20 minutes on medium, stirring occasionally. Add the curry and continue stirring.

2. Add the squash, broth, salt and 2 cups of water. Heat to a boil. Reduce to low and simmer for 30 minutes.

3. Place soup in a blender in small batches until smooth.

# Gazpacho

*Add Tabasco sauce if you prefer spicy gazpacho.*

1. Mix all ingredients together in a large pot. Combine thoroughly.

2. Transfer to a blender and blend in portions.

3. Refrigerate in bowls for 2–3 hours to chill.

### History of Gazpacho

Gazpacho is a cold Spanish soup, created for the summer to cool off during the hot, humid weather. It's traditionally made with tomatoes and served with hard-boiled eggs.

*Yields 8 servings*
Calories: 122
Fat: 7 grams
Protein: 3 grams
Carbohydrates: 15 grams
Cholesterol: 0 milligrams

*6 tomatoes, peeled and chopped*
*1 purple onion, finely chopped*
*1 seedless cucumber, chopped and peeled*
*1 green pepper, seeded and chopped*
*2 celery stalks, chopped*
*3 tablespoons parsley, chopped*
*2 tablespoons chives, chopped*
*1 clove garlic, crushed*
*¼ cup olive oil*
*3 tablespoons lemon juice*
*1 teaspoon sugar*
*salt and pepper to taste*
*4 cups tomato juice*

# Potato Mock Turtle Soup

*You can get fresh clam meat from your grocery fish market. Add 1 tablespoon
of sherry to each bowl to give the dish an extra flavor burst.*

**_Yields 4 servings_**
Calories: 75
Fat: 1 gram
Protein: 7 grams
Carbohydrates: 12 grams
Cholesterol: 14 millligrams

½ cup fresh clams
4 cups low-sodium chicken stock
1 potato, chopped into small chunks
1 bay leaf
1 teaspoon lemon juice
2 drops Tabasco sauce
salt and pepper to taste

1. Combine the clams, chicken stock, potato chunks, bay leaf, lemon juice, and Tabasco in a large pot; bring it to a boil.

2. Reduce heat to a simmer until clams are cooked to tender.

3. Remove bay leaf. Season with salt and pepper

## The Mock Turtle

The Mock Turtle is a fictional character in Lewis Carroll's book, *Alice's Adventures in Wonderland*. The character name was meant as a pun on the dish mock turtle soup, which was a popular Victorian delicacy that used parts of cattle that were not traditionally eaten.

# French Onion Soup

This soup is best with toasted French bread, but you can toast nearly any type of bread for dipping. Heat the bowls in the microwave and the cheese melts just as well as in the broiler.

1   Preheat broiler.

2.  In a large pot, cook the onions with the margarine until brown. Add the broth, Worcestershire sauce, and pepper; bring to a boil.

3.  Pour into individual ovenproof bowls. Top with toasted bread and grated cheese. Place under broiler and heat until cheese bubbles and serve.

## French Onion Soup

History tells us that French onion soup was created by King Louis XV of France. He wanted something to eat late one night but only had onions, butter, and champagne, so he mixed them together and the first French onion soup was born.

**Yields 8 servings**
Calories: 255
Fat: 6 grams
Protein: 12 grams
Carbohydrates: 38 grams
Cholesterol: 2 milligrams

2 large white onions, thinly sliced
2 tablespoons margarine
32 ounces low-sodium beef broth
2 tablespoons Worcestershire sauce
1 teaspoon freshly ground pepper
¾ cup nonfat grated cheese, any type
8 medium slices French bread, toasted

# Spiced Carrot Soup

*When you slice the carrots, slice them in circles, not long strips.*
*You can also serve this soup cold.*

### Yields 6 servings

Calories: 83
Fat: 3 grams
Protein: 2 grams
Carbohydrates: 15 grams
Cholesterol: 0 milligrams

6 carrots, thinly sliced
1 large onion, finely chopped
6 cups low-sodium chicken broth
1 tablespoon margarine
¼ teaspoon cumin
¼ teaspoon coriander
⅓ teaspoon cayenne pepper
1 teaspoon salt
1 teaspoon pepper

1. In a deep saucepan, simmer the carrots and onion with the chicken broth and margarine until the carrots are tender.

2. Remove carrots and onions to a blender. Puree the carrots and onion, then return to the saucepan.

3. Mix in the spices, salt and pepper and simmer for 30 minutes, then serve.

# Spicy Thai Beef Noodle Soup

*If you can't find rice noodles, vermicelli will do as well.*

1. Cut noodles into 3" pieces.

2. Heat the peanut oil in a deep saucepan over medium heat. Add jalapeño, and ginger. Sauté for 2 minutes.

3. Add the flank steak and sauté until browned throughout, stirring constantly.

4. Add the broth and soy sauce; bring to a boil. Reduce heat to medium; cover and simmer 10 minutes.

5. Add noodles and peas; simmer until noodles are tender, about 5 minutes. Add scallions, cilantro, and Tabasco sauce. Serve hot.

*Yields 4 servings*
Calories: 300
Fat: 7 grams
Protein: 17 grams
Carbohydrates: 40 grams
Cholesterol: 22 milligrams

1 6-ounce package rice noodles
2 teaspoons peanut oil
1 jalapeño pepper, seeded and minced
1 tablespoon ginger root, minced
6 ounces flank steak, sliced thinly across the grain
7 cups fat-free beef broth
2 tablespoons low-sodium soy sauce
½ cup green peas
4 scallions, chopped
2 tablespoons cilantro, chopped
1 teaspoon Tabasco sauce

# Black Bean Soup

*Serve with baked tortilla chips for a delicious meal.*

*Yields 4 servings*
Calories: 75
Fat: <1 gram
Protein: 5 grams
Carbohydrates: 17 grams
Cholesterol: 0 milligrams

*1 15-ounce can black beans, rinsed*
   *and drained*
*2 cups water*
*1 cup chopped tomatoes*
*1 teaspoon ground cumin*
*1 teaspoon sugar*
*¼ cup mild salsa*

1. Set aside 4 tablespoons of black beans to use later. Place beans, salsa, water, and tomato chunks in a large pot and mix. Mix in the cumin and sugar.

2. Place all ingredients in a blender in equal parts and puree until smooth. Place back into a large pot and heat on medium until bubbling. Serve hot and garnish with the remaining black beans.

## Black Beans

Black beans help lower cholesterol and are high in fiber, which helps slow rising blood sugar levels. Black beans are a particularly wise choice for people with diabetes or hypoglycemia. They are a virtually fat-free protein as well.

# Split Pea Soup

*You can add nearly any spice you want to this recipe.*

1. In a large pot, boil the water and add the peas, garlic, oregano, bay leaf, carrots, onion, and bouillon cubes.

2. Let boil for 30 minutes, then reduce to a simmer. Simmer for about 1 hour, stirring occasionally. Remove the bay leaf.

3. Transfer ingredients to a blender in portions and puree. Garnish with chopped onion.

*Yields 8 servings*
Calories: 215
Fat: <1 gram
Protein: 20 grams
Carbohydrates: 52 grams
Cholesterol: <1 milligram

*1 16-ounce package split peas*
*3 quarts water*
*1 clove garlic, crushed*
*1 teaspoon oregano*
*1 bay leaf*
*2 cubes chicken bouillon*
*3 carrots, chopped*
*1 purple onion, chopped*

# Cream of Mushroom Soup

## Yields 4 servings
Calories: 95
Fat: 4 grams
Protein: 5 grams
Carbohydrates: 11 grams
Cholesterol: 1 milligram

1 tablespoon margarine
2 cups mushrooms, chopped
1 onion, chopped
2 tablespoons flour
1 cup chicken broth
1 cup skim milk
¼ cup parsley, chopped

This soup can also be used as a base for casserole; it's particularly good with chicken casserole.

1. Melt the margarine in a large saucepan. Add the chopped mushrooms and onion; sauté over medium heat. Stir in the flour, then add the chicken broth. Simmer for 10 minutes.

2. Transfer to a blender in parts and puree.

3. Pour mixture back into saucepan and simmer for 15 minutes. Stir in the milk and chopped parsley. Simmer for 10 minutes and serve.

# Corn Chowder

*Add chopped celery, carrots, and onions to add some color to this delightful soup.*

1. Heat the olive oil in a deep saucepan over medium heat. Add the corn, potatoes, water, salt, and paprika; bring to a boil for 10 minutes. Reduce heat to medium and cook until potatoes are tender.

2. Put ½ cup of milk in a jar with a tight-fitting lid, add the flour, and shake vigorously.

3. Mix the milk and flour with cooked veggies. Add remaining milk, turn heat up, and stir. Bring mixture to a boil and continue stirring for five minutes.

4. Serve and garnish with fresh chopped parsley.

## Corn Chowder

Corn chowder developed from clam chowder, replacing clams with corn and sometimes bacon bits. It is typically made with heavy cream, but substituting skim milk keeps the calories down.

*Yields 4 servings*
Calories: 174
Fat: 5 grams
Protein: 7 grams
Carbohydrates: 29 grams
Cholesterol: 3 milligrams

*1 tablespoon olive oil*
*1 10-ounce package whole kernel corn*
*1 cup potato, cut into chunks*
*1 cup water*
*¼ teaspoon salt*
*¼ teaspoon paprika*
*2 tablespoons flour*
*2 cups skim milk*
*2 tablespoons parsley, chopped*

# Creamy Potato Soup

*This is another soup that is great as a puree. Place everything in a blender,
one cup at a time, and serve after blending to a creamy consistency.*

*Yields 4 servings*
Calories: 395
Fat: 6 grams
Protein: 16 grams
Carbohydrates: 70 grams
Cholesterol: 16 milligrams

*16 ounces low-sodium cream of
    chicken soup
6 red potatoes, chopped
1 onion, chopped
2½ cups skim milk
1 teaspoon dried dill weed
pepper to taste*

1. Bring the chicken soup and potatoes to a boil in a large pot and cook for 20 minutes.

2. Add the chopped onion and turn heat down to medium. Add the skim milk and cook for 30 minutes.

3. Reduce to a simmer, and add in the dill weed. Stir for 5 minutes and serve. Sprinkle pepper over each bowl of soup.

## Stone Soup Fable

Three weary travelers arrived in a village with nothing but a soup kettle. They asked the villagers to share their food, but the villagers refused. "No matter," said one of the travelers, and he filled the kettle with water, added a stone, and put the whole thing over a fire to cook. One by one, curious villagers asked what the travelers were doing. "We're making stone soup," the travelers replied. "It's delicious, but it would be perfect if we just had some . . ." And so the villagers were tricked into sharing their food. Before long, the travelers had a delicious soup simmering away.

# 10

# Beef and Pork

# Super-Skinny Skillet Beef Stew

*This is a great dish that can be served alone or over a bed of rice or noodles.*

*Yields 4 servings*
Calories: 385
Fat: 17 grams
Protein: 38 grams
Carbohydrates: 20 grams
Cholesterol: 115 milligrams

*1 tablespoon olive oil*
*1 pound lean beef stew meat, cut into 1" cubes*
*1 large onion, cut into small cubes*
*2 medium carrots, thickly sliced*
*2 cloves garlic, chopped*
*1 15-ounce can tomatoes*
*1 cup canned beef broth*
*2 tablespoons dried oregano*
*1 tablespoon salt*
*1 tablespoon Splenda*
*3 tablespoons Worcestershire sauce*

1. Heat olive oil in a heavy skillet. Brown beef cubes.

2. Add onions and carrots to skillet and sauté until soft.

3. Add the remaining ingredients; cover and let simmer for 1 hour.

4. Uncover and let simmer for 5 minutes.

## Savor the Juices

You can also combine all ingredients in a slow cooker and cook until the meat is tender. This is a nice option because you can let it cook all day so the juices soak in. As it cooks, the aroma of cooking beef fills your house so you can enjoy your meal before you eat it.

# Beef Stir Fry

*Prepare this recipe in a wok. That way the heat is distributed evenly, making it virtually goof-proof.*

1. Heat the peanut oil in a heavy skillet or wok.

2. Add the ginger root and chili peppers.

3. Add sliced beef, soy sauce, Splenda, and cooking wine.

4. Stir ingredients until color of beef changes to brown.

## Asian Ingredients

Paper-thin slices of pre-prepared beef, ginger root, and shredded chili peppers can be purchased at most Asian markets. They are a good place to find herbs, spices, and produce to experiment with that you can't find at your regular market, and they also have wide selections of commonly used ingredients such as soy sauce.

*Yields 4 servings*
Calories: 255
Fat: 21 grams
Protein: 12 grams
Carbohydrates: 4 grams
Cholesterol: 38 milligrams

3 tablespoons peanut oil
2 tablespoons shredded ginger root
½ cup shredded red hot chili peppers
½ pound sliced beef
3 tablespoons soy sauce
1 tablespoon Splenda
1 tablespoon red cooking wine

# Beef Chili

***Yields 4 servings***
Calories: 385
Fat: 10 grams
Protein: 35 grams
Carbohydrates: 37 grams
Cholesterol: 70 milligrams

*3 cloves garlic, minced*
*1 tablespoon canola oil*
*1 pound lean ground beef*
*1 15-ounce can tomatoes*
*1 16-ounce can red kidney beans*
*½ teaspoon cumin seed*
*½ teaspoon oregano*
*1½ tablespoons chili powder*
*salt and pepper to taste*

*Serve this beef chili in oversized mugs and garnish with low-fat shredded cheese and a dollop of nonfat sour cream. It makes an especially cozy dish on cold winter nights.*

1. Sauté garlic in the canola oil in a heavy skillet over medium heat.

2. Add the ground beef, mixing thoroughly until meat is brown.

3. Reduce heat to low. Add the tomatoes and beans, mixing thoroughly.

4. Add the cumin, oregano, chili powder, salt, and pepper.

5. Cover and simmer for 1 hour, stirring occasionally.

# Beef Tenderloin

This recipe is as simple as it is tasty—in a word, extremely. You can add as much dry sherry as you like and it can only enhance the flavors in the meat.

1. Preheat oven to 400°F.

2. Trim fat off of the tenderloin.

3. Place tenderloin into a shallow baking pan and bake for 10 minutes.

4. In a skillet, sauté the onion in the olive oil over medium heat. Add the sherry, soy sauce, mustard, salt, and pepper. Bring to a boil.

5. Pour the mixture over the tenderloin and reduce oven temperature to 325°F for 20 minutes, basting occasionally. Serve tenderloin with drippings.

*Yields 4 servings*
Calories: 320
Fat: 22 grams
Protein: 26 grams
Carbohydrates: 2 grams
Cholesterol: 77 milligrams

*1 pound beef tenderloin*
*¼ cup olive oil*
*¼ cup chopped onion*
*½ cup dry sherry*
*1 tablespoon lite soy sauce*
*1 teaspoon dry mustard*
*salt and pepper to taste*

# Beef Fajitas

*You can serve these fajitas in corn or flour tortillas or over a bed of rice. Add pico de gallo to your liking.*

***Yields 4 servings***
Calories: 610
Fat: 26 grams
Protein: 31 grams
Carbohydrates: 58 grams
Cholesterol: 45 milligrams

*1 pound extra lean beef round
    steaks, cut into thin strips
1 envelope fajita seasoning mix
1 small onion, diced
1 green bell pepper, sliced
1 small red bell pepper, sliced
½ cup water
1 11-ounce packet corn tortillas*

1. Sprinkle steak strips with fajita seasoning in a medium bowl, making sure to cover all sides.

2. Sauté onion and peppers in heavy skillet until soft.

3. Add steak to vegetables and add water.

4. Cover and simmer for 3–4 hours.

5. Serve with tortillas (or over rice).

## Sauté Tips

When you sauté multiple ingredients and liquids on the stove, you need to make sure you use a skillet or frying pan with high sides, at least about 1½", to minimize splatter. A splatter screen is also a good investment. Not only does splattered oil make a mess of your stovetop and clothes, it hurts when it hits your skin!

# Beef Fondue

Select a variety of sauces, like barbeque, mustard, or sweet and sour sauce, to dip your beef in after cooking.

1. Heat oil in fondue pot until it boils.

2. Dip each cube in hot oil until cooked.

3. Choose your sauce flavor and enjoy.

_Yields 4 servings_
Calories: 615
Fat: 60 grams
Protein: 22 grams
Carbohydrates: 0 grams
Cholesterol: 60 milligrams

1 pound filet mignon, cut into 1"
    cubes
1 cup canola oil
fondue pot and skewers
3 tablespoons each of a variety of
    sauces

# Flank Steak

*Flank steak is most flavorful when cooked to medium, a little pink in the middle.*

**Yields 4 servings**
Calories: 448
Fat: 28 grams
Protein: 48 grams
Carbohydrates: 2 grams
Cholesterol: 76 milligrams

*1 teaspoon salt*
*1 teaspoon coarse ground black*
*    pepper*
*1½ pounds flank steak*
*1 clove garlic, chopped*
*¼ cup garlic-flavored olive oil*
*6 tablespoons cider vinegar*
*2 teaspoons soy sauce*

1.  Sprinkle salt and pepper liberally on both sides of steak.

2.  Make small slits with sharp knife over steak on both sides so the salt and pepper can soak in and season the meat.

3.  Place all other ingredients in a plastic bag, seal, and shake well.

4.  Add the flank steak to the plastic bag and let it sit for 2–6 hours.

5.  Transfer flank steak to grill and cook to desired doneness.

6.  Transfer steak to cutting board and slice diagonally across the grain, making very thin slices, about ⅛" thick.

# Beef Satay

*You can add any type of vegetable to these to top them off.*

1. Thread beef chunks onto skewers.

2. Mix the yogurt, garlic, curry powder, and lemon juice together in a small bowl.

3. Coat the beef skewers with the yogurt mixture.

4. Place skewers with beef and marinade into the refrigerator for several hours to let the marinade soak in.

5. Grill beef satays until tender.

## Grilling with Skewers

Soak your wooden skewers in water before you grill with them to avoid any undesirable fires. Dry wooden skewers have been known to catch fire, a potential threat to you and your food. To make sure your skewers don't get weighed down with the meat, use two skewers per kabob.

<u>*Yields 4 servings*</u>
Calories: 328
Fat: 22 grams
Protein: 26 grams
Carbohydrates: 6 grams
Cholesterol: 79 milligrams

*1 pound beef tenderloin, cut into 2"
    strips
15–20 wooden skewers, soaked in
    water for 20 minutes
1 cup plain nonfat yogurt
1 teaspoon minced garlic
2 teaspoons curry powder
juice of 1 lemon*

# Corned Beef and Cabbage

*This meal can be easily prepared on the stovetop in a large pot.*

## Yields 4 servings
Calories: 680
Fat: 34 grams
Protein: 41 grams
Carbohydrates: 53 grams
Cholesterol: 123 milligrams

1–2 pounds corned beef brisket
2 large potatoes, peeled and
    quartered
3 carrots, peeled and quartered
2 onions, quartered
1 small head cabbage, cut into large
    pieces

1. Place the corned beef in a deep roasting pan or heavy pot and cover with water.

2. Bring water to boil, then simmer for 1 hour, adding water if necessary.

3. Add vegetables, cutting cabbage into large pieces.

4. Return to a boil, reduce heat, and simmer for 20 minutes until vegetables are cooked.

5. Remove from heat, cool, and slice corned beef across the grain.

## Corned Beef Tradition

Corned beef is very popular on St. Patrick's Day. Irish-Americans like to eat corned beef and cabbage to celebrate the holiday. It's one of the dishes most associated with Irish cuisine, but interestingly it isn't a national favorite in Ireland itself.

The Everything Calorie Counting Cookbook

# Roast Beef

You can add literally anything to the meat while roasting. Some suggestions
to consider: potatoes, carrots, onions, garlic, and red wine.

1. Preheat oven to 325°F.

2. Rub roast with the salt and Splenda brown sugar.

3. Put roast beef in roasting pan. Add ¼ cup water to pan.

4. Cook for about 3 hours or until tender.

## Shakespeare's Roast Beef

The popularity of beef in English culture is alluded to in Shakespeare's *Henry V.* "Give them
great meals of beef and iron and steel, they will eat like wolves and fight like devils." (Act 3,
Scene 7) In England, roast beef is often eaten with Yorkshire pudding, which is like a popover,
and beans and bacon.

_Yields 4 servings_
Calories: 605
Fat: 40 grams
Protein: 59 grams
Carbohydrates: 15 grams
Cholesterol: 180 grams

1–2 pounds beef roast
1 teaspoon seasoned salt
2 tablespoons Splenda brown sugar
¼ cup water

# Beef Tacos

_Yields 4 servings_
Calories: 483
Fat: 19 grams
Protein: 45 grams
Carbohydrates: 29 grams
Cholesterol: 106 milligrams

1 pound extra lean ground beef
1 tablespoon canola oil
1 1.25-ounce packet low-sodium
    taco seasoning mix
8 hard taco shells
4 ounces shredded Mexican cheese
½ head lettuce, shredded
1 tomato, diced
1 small onion, diced
½ cup nonfat sour cream

1. Brown ground beef in canola oil until thoroughly cooked.

2. Mix taco seasoning with ground beef and water to taste.

3. Warm taco shells in oven at 325°F for 10 minutes.

4. Spoon seasoned meat into warm taco shell.

5. Layer the rest of the ingredients on top of meat as desired.

# Prime Rib of Beef

To lower the fat content of your roast, trim the fat before seasoning.

1. Preheat oven to 350°F.

2. Rub garlic powder, salt, and black pepper over the roast, massaging as you go.

3. Place roast, onion, celery, and beef broth into roasting pan.

4. Bake uncovered for 2–3 hours. Skim fat from pan drippings and serve.

## And How Would You Like That Cooked?

When roasting meat, use a meat thermometer to check the internal temperature to cook according to how you like your meat. For rare meat, the thermometer should read 125°F, medium 135°F, medium well 145°F, and well done 155°F to 160°F.

*Yields 10 servings; serving size 9 ounces*
Calories: 455
Fat: 39 grams
Protein: 23 grams
Carbohydrates: 2 grams
Cholesterol: 97 milligrams

*1 3-pound beef rib roast*
*½ teaspoon garlic powder*
*salt and pepper to taste*
*1 small onion, chopped*
*3 stalks celery, chopped*
*1 14-ounce can low-sodium beef broth*

# Beef Stroganoff

**Yields 4 servings**
Calories: 488
Fat: 22 grams
Protein: 33 grams
Carbohydrates: 38 grams
Cholesterol: 69 milligrams

¼ cup canola oil
1 large onion, finely chopped
1 clove garlic, finely chopped
1 pound very lean flank steak
2 cups mushrooms, sliced
1 tablespoon corn starch
2 tablespoons cooking sherry
1 cup low-sodium beef broth
salt and pepper to taste
1 cup fat-free sour cream
2 cups cooked wide noodles
½ cup parsley, finely chopped

*If you like, substitute 1–2 cups of cooked rice for the noodles.*

1. Thinly slice steak.

2. Sauté onions and garlic in canola oil over medium heat. Add steak and mushrooms. Cook until meat is tender.

3. Mix cornstarch, sherry, and broth in a small bowl to make a paste. Pour paste into meat mixture and let simmer for 5 minutes. Add salt, pepper, and sour cream.

4. Pour over hot noodles. Garnish with parsley.

## Brief Beef Stroganoff History

This dish dates back to medieval Russia. It was very popular in American homes in the 1950s because it is a very simple and filling meal that can be easily made in large quantities.

# Beef and Vegetable Cheese Casserole

*If you want to add noodles, try mixing in 1 cup of whole wheat pasta or noodles.*

1. Heat oil in a skillet. Brown the onions. Add ground beef.

2. While beef cooks, microwave mixed vegetables until thawed.

3. Drain fat from fully browned beef. Add vegetables and nonfat sour cream to the skillet. Mix well.

4. Pour into a casserole dish and sprinkle with low-fat cheddar cheese.

## The Medieval Casserole

A casserole is a dish or pot that is ideal for slow cooking many different foods together. A medieval casserole was a pastry filled with meats and spices and slowly cooked. Today, casseroles have expanded to include vegetables and bread crumbs, as well as many other ingredients.

**_Yields 4 servings_**
Calories: 398
Fat: 17 grams
Protein: 42 grams
Carbohydrates: 17 grams
Cholesterol: 83 milligrams

2 tablespoons canola oil
1 medium onion, chopped
1 pound lean ground beef
1 9-ounce bag frozen mixed
    vegetables
½ cup nonfat sour cream
8 ounces 2 percent shredded low-fat
    cheddar cheese

# Cola Pork Chops

**Yields 4 servings**
Calories: 213
Fat: 11 grams
Protein: 21 grams
Carbohydrates: 6 grams
Cholesterol: 59 milligrams

4 pork chops, fat removed
salt and pepper to taste
1 cup low-carb catsup
1 cup diet cola
1 tablespoon Splenda brown sugar

This is a uniquely delicious recipe. The soda does not yield enough calories to impact the recipe, so you can use regular soda if you prefer.

1. Preheat oven to 350°F.

2. Place the pork chops in a baking pan. Season pork chops with salt and pepper to taste.

3. Mix the catsup with the cola and pour over the pork chops. Sprinkle chops with Splenda brown sugar.

4. Bake for 1 hour or until pork chops are tender.

# BBQ Pork Sandwich

*To cut calories, eat the pulled pork without the buns or on a bed of lettuce.*

1. Make shallow slits in the skin of the roast. Stick whole cloves into the roast and rub it with barbeque seasoning.

2. Put the roast in to a slow cooker and top with onion slices.

3. Cover with water and slow cook for 8 hours.

4. Remove pork from crock pot and remove cloves from pork.

5. When pork cools, pull the meat apart with your fingers.

6. Return pulled meat to crock pot and add barbeque sauce.

7. Heat on low heat for 1 hour.

8. Serve over low-carb hamburger buns.

## Pulled Pork's Roots

Pigs were more abundant than cattle in the colonial American South, and therefore the early settlers ate more pork than beef. Pulled pork has evolved to become a barbecue classic. Letting the pork simmer for 8 hours loosens the meat, and it falls easily into pieces when you pull on it.

*Yields 4 servings*
Calories: 618
Fat: 21 grams
Protein: 61 grams
Carbohydrates: 45 grams
Cholesterol: 109 milligrams

*2 pounds pork shoulder roast, fat removed*
*3–4 whole cloves*
*2 tablespoons barbeque seasoning*
*1 large red onion, sliced*
*1 cup water*
*8 ounces barbeque sauce*
*4 low-carb hamburger buns*

# Garlic Pork Loin

*Garlic and rosemary provide classic seasoning for this low-calorie dish.*

**Yields 4 servings**
Calories: 330
Fat: 10 grams
Protein: 49 grams
Carbohydrates: 9 grams
Cholesterol: 143 milligrams

1 packet dry onion soup mix
2-pound pork roast, fat removed
1 teaspoon fresh rosemary
2 crushed garlic cloves
1 teaspoon dry mustard
1 teaspoon marjoram leaves

1. Line a shallow baking pan with heavy-duty aluminum foil.

2. Sprinkle onion soup mix on the bottom of the pan. Place roast on top of soup mix. Sprinkle rosemary, garlic, mustard, and marjoram on top of roast. Cover roast with aluminum foil.

3. Bake at 300°F for 3½–4 hours or until completely done.

# Mamma's Pork Chops

*The key to good pork chops is making sure you drain them thoroughly when you brown them. This will keep them from being greasy.*

**Yields 4 servings**
Calories: 510
Fat: 34 grams
Protein: 35 grams
Carbohydrates: 17 grams
Cholesterol: 111 milligrams

4 6-ounce pork chops, fat removed
2 tablespoons canola oil
½ cup cooked rice
1 10-ounce can cream of mushroom
   soup
1 cup light sour cream

1. Brown chops with canola oil and drain.

2. Place rice in a baking dish and top with the pork chops.

3. Mix the soup and sour cream together. Pour over the pork chops.

4. Bake at 350°F for 45 minutes.

# 11

# Fish

# Tuna Burgers

*Yields 6 servings*
Calories: 464
Fat: 12 grams
Protein: 58 grams
Carbohydrates: 28 grams
Cholesterol: 101 milligrams

3 6-ounce cans low-sodium tuna
4 tablespoons sweet pickle relish
½ cup chopped celery
4 tablespoons chopped onions
3 tablespoons light mayonnaise
3 low-carb hamburger buns

If you like cheese on your burger, add a slice of low-fat cheese to
each tuna burger before you broil so it melts nicely into the tuna.

1. Preheat the broiler.

2. Mix the tuna, relish, celery, onion, and mayonnaise in a medium bowl.

3. Spread tuna mixture on top of hamburger bun halves.

4. Assemble buns on a cookie sheet evenly and broil until bread toasts.

# Tuna Casserole

*You can replace the cream of chicken soup with cream of mushroom
if you prefer, just be sure to keep it low sodium.*

1. Preheat oven to 400°F.

2. Mix the soup and milk together in a small bowl.

3. In a medium bowl, mix the noodles, green beans, tuna, and pepper, then add the soup/milk mixture and gently fold.

4. Pour everything into a baking dish and cover with foil.

5. Bake until the casserole starts to bubble, about 25 minutes. Uncover and sprinkle crumbs on top. Bake uncovered until crumbs are browned.

**Yields 4 servings**
Calories: 278
Fat: 7 grams
Protein: 19 grams
Carbohydrates: 37 grams
Cholesterol: 24 milligrams

1 10-ounce can low-sodium cream
    of chicken soup
½ cup fat-free milk
2 cups cooked whole wheat
    macaroni noodles
10 ounces frozen cut green beans
1 6-ounce can tuna, drained
¼ teaspoon freshly ground black
    pepper
5 tablespoons bread crumbs

# Grilled Tuna with Vegetables

*You can use any type of oil-based salad dressing or plain olive oil for the marinade.*

*Yields 4 servings*
Calories: 475
Fat: 13 grams
Protein: 76 grams
Carbohydrates: 10 grams
Cholesterol: 160 milligrams

*1 cup light Italian dressing*
*4 cloves garlic, crushed*
*1 onion, finely chopped or grated*
*4 12-ounce tuna steaks*

1. Mix dressing, garlic, and onion in a medium bowl.

2. Pour mixture into 4 separate large resealable plastic bags. Place one steak into each bag and let each marinate in the mixture for about 2 hours.

3. Turn on grill and let it heat up.

4. Place each fillet on the hottest part of the grill for about 3 minutes each side.

### Grilling Tuna

Whether you have an electric, gas, or traditional charcoal grill, make sure the grill is nice and hot before you put the tuna steaks on. Tuna can be served with a little pink inside if you prefer your steaks rare; an opaque color means it's well done. Cut on the side to test as you grill.

# Pan-Fried Salmon

*You can pan-fry salmon fillets with or without the skin depending on what you like. When cooking the side with skin, allow salmon to cook a little longer.*

*Yields 4 servings*
Calories: 685
Fat: 39 grams
Protein: 79 grams
Carbohydrates: 1 gram
Cholesterol: 218 milligrams

*4 tablespoons olive oil*
*1 large lemon*
*4 8-ounce salmon fillets*
*salt and pepper to taste*

1. Heat olive oil in a large skillet on medium heat.

2. Squeeze lemon liberally over salmon fillets on all sides.

3. Season fish with salt and pepper and place on pan.

4. Cook fish on both sides until it browns.

### Choosing Salmon Fillets

You want to purchase a salmon fillet that is about 1" thick, preferably a center cut. Salmon is naturally a rich pink color. The larger the fish, the more likely you will find bones in a fillet. Before cooking, hold a pair of pliers and run the finger of your other hand down the fillet, against the grain. Whenever you feel a bone, press down close to it. It will pop up, and you can then pull it out with the pliers.

# Salmon Loaf

*This is a twist on traditional meatloaf and a delightful low-calorie,
low-fat treat to serve your family with a side of green beans.*

1.  Preheat oven to 350°F

2.  Heat the olive oil in a skillet over medium heat. Sauté the shallots until tender.

3.  In a large bowl, mix the shallots, cracker crumbs, milk, egg, and lemon juice. Beat well. Add salmon to the bowl and mix well.

4.  Lightly spray a baking pan. Place salmon mixture in the baking pan and bake for about 1 hour or until brown.

*Yields 8 servings*
Calories: 196
Fat: 11 grams
Protein: 12 grams
Carbohydrates: 11 grams
Cholesterol: 54 milligrams

*2 tablespoons olive oil*
*½ cup chopped shallots*
*½ cup light Ritz crackers, crushed*
*½ cup fat-free milk*
*1 egg, beaten*
*4 teaspoons lemon juice*
*1 14-ounce can salmon*
*light cooking spray*

# Salmon with Dill

*Serve these steaks for a Fourth of July barbecue, along
with some potato salad and grilled corn on the cob.*

1.  In a mini food processor, coffee grinder, or with a mortar and pestle, grind dill seed with salt and pepper until very fine. Sprinkle on both sides of salmon steaks. Place salmon in a large glass baking dish. In small bowl, combine orange juice, lemon juice, and olive oil; pour over salmon. Cover and refrigerate for 1 hour.

2.  When ready to cook, prepare and preheat grill. Remove salmon from marinade. Grill salmon 6" over medium coals until desired doneness (3 to 5 minutes for rare, 5 to 8 minutes for medium, 8 to 10 minutes for well done), turning once. Brush salmon with remaining marinade as it grills (discard unused marinade). Serve immediately.

*Yields 4 servings*
Calories: 323
Fat: 18 grams
Protein: 64 grams
Carbohydrates: 2 grams
Cholesterol: 106 milligrams

*1 teaspoon dill seed*
*½ teaspoon salt*
*⅛ teaspoon white pepper*
*4 salmon steaks*
*¼ cup orange juice*
*1 tablespoon lemon juice*
*2 tablespoons olive oil*

# Fettuccini with Salmon

To keep the fettuccine noodles from sticking together when you cook
them, add a capful of olive oil to the boiling water and stir the noodles often.

**Yields 4 servings**
Calories: 650
Fat: 13 grams
Protein: 43 grams
Grams of Carbohydrates: 91
grams
Cholesterol: 65 milligrams

1 tablespoon olive oil
¼ cup white wine
salt and pepper to taste
1 pound salmon fillet
1 onion, chopped
1 teaspoon flour
2 cups skim milk
1 pound spinach fettuccine
¼ cup olive oil
2 tablespoons dill
2 tablespoons lemon juice

1. Mix the wine, 1 tablespoon olive oil, and seasonings in a deep skillet and bring them to a boil.

2. Cut the salmon into 4 pieces and add to skillet. Cook for 3 minutes on each side.

3. Remove salmon to a plate and cover with foil.

4. Stir onion in the skillet and cook for about 5 minutes.

5. Add flour and skim milk, stirring constantly while it thickens.

6. Turn heat off. Cover and set aside.

7. Cook fettuccini in boiling water for about 3 minutes.

8. Meanwhile, heat ¼ cup olive oil in a small skillet.

9. Add the dill and lemon to the olive oil. Mix well, then remove from heat and set aside.

10. Drain pasta, place it in a medium bowl, and toss with the olive oil mixture.

11. Place the salmon back in skillet and simmer over medium heat for about 5 minutes.

12. Serve salmon on a plate of pasta and spoon sauce on top.

The Everything Calorie Counting Cookbook

# Zesty Crumb-Coated Cod

Instead of a slice of bread, you can crush croutons to make crumbs and add those to the food processor. This recipe is ideal for bread products that are slightly stale.

1. Preheat the broiler.

2. Squeeze 2 tablespoons of lemon juice into a food processor. Place bread in the food processor and pulse until crumbs form.

3. Place cod in a baking pan and squeeze lemon over to your liking. Sprinkle cod with salt and pepper. Pat cod fillet with the bread crumbs, turning fillet so you get both sides.

4. Broil for about 8 minutes or until crumbs turn golden.

*Yields 3 servings*
Calories: 153
Fat: 1 gram
Protein: 28 grams
Carbohydrates: 6 grams
Cholesterol: 65 milligrams

*1 lemon*
*1 slice whole wheat bread*
*1 pound cod fillet*
*salt and pepper to taste*

# Oven-Fried Fish

Any mild, white fish is a great choice for this recipe. In addition to cod,
haddock and tilapia work particularly well.

**Yields 4 servings**
Calories: 215
Fat: 7 grams
Protein: 25 grams
Carbohydrates: 13 grams
Cholesterol: 118 milligrams

1 egg
½ teaspoon salt
½ teaspoon pepper
4 4-ounce cod fillets
2 tablespoons flour
½ cup bread crumbs
1 tablespoon olive oil

1. Preheat oven to 500°F.

2. Beat the egg, salt, and pepper in a small bowl. Dredge both sides of the fish in flour. Dip fillets in beaten egg mixture. Pat bread crumbs over moist fillets until coated. Place coated fish on baking pan and drizzle olive oil over each piece.

3. Bake for 20 minutes or until fillets are crisp and golden.

### Fish in the Food Pyramid
New dietary guidelines recommend increased variation in adult diets. Beef and poultry make up the bulk of meat sales, but fish are high in beneficial oils and fats. Fish contain monounsaturated fatty acids and polyunsaturated fatty acids, which should account for most of a healthy adult's fat intake.

# Grilled Halibut with Vegetables

You can grill literally any vegetable with this recipe. It is best to use a vegetable skillet designed for grills, as they have holes and allow air to travel through the skillet so your veggies don't burn.

**Yields 4 servings**
Calories: 290
Fat: 17 grams
Protein: 28 grams
Carbohydrates: 9 grams
Cholesterol: 36 milligrams

1 10-ounce can low-sodium chicken
    broth
3 tablespoons lemon juice
4 tablespoons olive oil
4 4-ounce halibut steaks
1 red pepper, cut in quarters
1 green pepper, cut in quarters
14 ounces frozen broccoli

1. Mix chicken broth, lemon juice, and olive oil in a medium bowl.

2. Brush each halibut streak with the chicken broth mixture on both sides.

3. Heat grill to medium and place steaks on grill, turning every 3 minutes until done.

4. Add vegetables to a vegetable pan over grill, tossing gently as they cook.

5. Serve vegetables and halibut together.

# Herb and Lemon Baked Halibut

You can add any herbs you like to this recipe. Experiment with fresh and dried herbs, but remember that dried herbs are concentrated so you will need fewer of them.

1. Preheat oven to 375°F.

2. Place the lemon slices in a baking pan.

3. Rub the fish on both sides with olive oil, salt, pepper, parsley, basil, and thyme.

4. Place the halibut over the lemons and bake for about 20 minutes or until the fish flakes and cooks through.

## Cooking with Herbs

You can add any herbs or seasonings you want to a recipe to give it your signature. Halibut live in northern waters; most dishes that feature halibut also showcase herbs common to northern areas, and this recipe is no exception. Play around with different flavors from more temperate climates, and try adding some spice.

*Yields 4 servings*
Calories: 168
Fat: 6 grams
Protein: 24 grams
Carbohydrates: 4 grams
Cholesterol: 36 milligrams

*2 lemons, sliced*
*1 pound fresh halibut*
*1 tablespoon olive oil*
*salt and pepper to taste*
*½ cup chopped parsley*
*2 tablespoons chopped basil*
*2 tablespoons thyme*

# Baked Halibut with Homemade Tartar Sauce

There's truly nothing tastier than homemade tartar sauce. You can make a larger batch and save it for your dishes throughout the week.

1. Preheat oven to 375°F.

2. Rub halibut with the oil. Squeeze lemon liberally over halibut. Place halibut in oven and bake for 20 minutes.

3. While halibut is baking, combine mayonnaise, mustard, dill pickle, parsley, shallots, capers, lemon juice, salt, and pepper in a medium bowl until smooth.

4. When halibut is ready, place a dollop of tartar sauce over each piece and serve.

*Yields 4 servings*
Calories: 293
Fat: 19 grams
Protein: 24 grams
Carbohydrates: 5 grams
Cholesterol: 46 milligrams

*1 pound fresh halibut*
*2 tablespoons olive oil*
*1 lemon*
*½ cup light mayonnaise*
*½ teaspoon Dijon mustard*
*1 tablespoon dill pickle, minced*
*1 tablespoon parsley, chopped*
*1 tablespoon shallots, chopped*
*2 teaspoons capers, chopped*
*1 teaspoon lemon juice*
*salt and pepper*

# Sautéed Halibut

*If the skillet gets dry, add more wine, lemon juice, or olive oil.*

1. Heat olive oil, wine, and lemon juice in a deep skillet over medium heat.

2. Add halibut and sauté until done.

## Funky Halibut Facts

Halibut is a member of the flounder family, and it is the largest of all the flat fish. Halibut can grow to be nearly 600 pounds. When the halibut is born it has eyes on both sides of its head, but as it matures one eye rotates to the other side of its head.

*Yields 4 servings*
Calories: 175
Fat: 7 grams
Protein: 23 grams
Carbohydrates: 3 grams
Cholesterol: 36 milligrams

*4 teaspoons olive oil*
*¼ cup dry white wine*
*2 tablespoons lemon juice*
*1 pound halibut*

# Baked Sole

*Baked sole goes well with rich pasta or baked potatoes, and greens.*

1. Preheat oven to 400°F.

2. Combine eggs, milk, and salt in small bowl.

3. Dip the sole in the egg mixture and then roll in bread crumbs.

4. Place breaded sole on a baking sheet and bake for 20 minutes or until fish flakes.

5. Sprinkle fillets with fresh lemon juice to taste.

*Yields 4 servings*
Calories: 255
Fat: 14 grams
Protein: 36 grams
Carbohydrates: 17 grams
Cholesterol: 131 milligrams

*1 egg, well beaten*
*¼ cup skim milk*
*½ teaspoon salt*
*4 4-ounce sole fillets*
*¾ cup bread crumbs*
*1 lemon*

# Tomato and Tarragon Sole

You can replace the canned tomatoes with simple low-sodium tomato soup if you prefer.

1. Preheat oven to 400°F.

2. Rub olive oil on sole fillets. Sprinkle fresh tarragon on sole fillets.

3. Pour tomatoes and juice in a baking dish. Place fillets in dish and bake for 30 minutes or until fish flakes.

## Tarragon Trivia
Tarragon is very common in French cooking and best used with fish or chicken. It is also one of the main ingredients in Béarnaise sauce. It has a very distinctive anise flavor that can easily overwhelm blander dishes, so be careful not to go overboard.

*Yields 4 servings*
Calories: 285
Fat: 16 grams
Protein: 32 grams
Carbohydrates: 4 grams
Cholesterol: 79 milligrams

*4 tablespoons olive oil*
*4 tablespoons fresh tarragon*
*4 4-ounce sole fillets*
*1 10-ounce can tomatoes in juice*

# Cuban-Style Braised Fish

Sprinkle pecans or almonds over the fish when it is done and serve with a side of vegetables.

1. Heat the olive oil in a large deep skillet over medium heat.

2. Add the onion and garlic and sauté for 5 minutes.

3. Add the tomatoes, jalepeños, chicken broth, and olives. Let simmer.

4. Add halibut and cook until fish flakes, about 10 minutes.

## Cuban Cuisine
Cuban cuisine has been influenced over centuries by Spanish, French, African, Arabic, Chinese, and Portuguese cultures. Most Cuban food is sautéed or slow-cooked over a low flame. Sofrito is a traditional seasoning; it consists of onion, green pepper, garlic, oregano, and ground pepper quick-fried in olive oil. Tomato-based sauces are also traditional in Cuban cooking.

*Yields 4 servings*
Calories: 223
Fat: 10 grams
Protein: 26 grams
Carbohydrates: 8 grams
Cholesterol: 36 milligrams

*2 teaspoons olive oil*
*1 onion, chopped*
*2 cloves garlic, diced*
*4 tomatoes, diced*
*3 jalapeños, diced*
*¾ cup low-sodium chicken broth*
*½ cup olives, thinly sliced*
*1 pound halibut*

# Lime-Seared Scallops

**Yields 4 servings**
Calories: 238
Fat: 6 grams
Protein: 31 grams
Carbohydrates: 19 grams
Cholesterol: 56 milligrams

*4 teaspoons olive oil, divided*
*1½ pounds scallops*
*2 teaspoons minced garlic*
*2 small shallots, chopped*
*2 limes*

*Scallops are usually prepared medium, a little tender inside, but if you prefer your scallops well done, keep searing to your taste and they will be slightly tougher throughout.*

1. In a deep skillet, heat 2 teaspoons olive oil for 4 minutes.

2. Drain juices from scallops and pat dry with a paper towel.

3. Add the scallops and sear them on each side for about 3 minutes, until scallops have a golden brown texture.

4. Remove scallops from skillet and set aside in a bowl.

5. Mix 2 teaspoons olive oil, garlic, shallots, and juice from 1 lime in a small bowl.

6. Pour lime marinade over scallops, mixing lightly with a wooden spoon.

7. Place scallops in the fridge for about 1 hour to marinate. Serve cold or heat up in microwave.

### Shopping for the Perfect Scallop

When purchasing scallops, note that "dry packed" scallops are additive free, while "wet packed" scallops contain sodium tripolyphosphate (STP), a salt-based preservative that causes the scallops to absorb water. This means they are bloated and the seller gets a better price per pound.

# Chili-Crusted Sea Scallops

*If you like it hot, you'll love these. These are true Cajun scallops!*

1. Preheat boiler. Spray baking sheet with light cooking spray.

2. Mix the lemon juice, chili powder, cumin, and cayenne pepper in a small saucepan over medium heat and let simmer about 3 minutes.

3. Drain scallops and transfer to a medium bowl. Pour mixture from saucepan over scallops and toss gently with a wooden spoon.

4. Evenly distribute scallops onto a baking sheet. Broil 20 minutes or until scallops are opaque.

## Scallops and Spinach
Scallops are great served over a bed of sautéed spinach. You can heat 4 tablespoons olive oil over medium heat, add 1 bag of prepackaged spinach, and sauté until soft. Serve the scallops over spinach.

*Yields 4 servings*
Calories: 65
Fat: 1 grams
Protein: 10 grams
Carbohydrates: 5 grams
Cholesterol: 18 grams

*light cooking spray*
*4 tablespoons lemon juice*
*2 teaspoons chili powder*
*½ teaspoon ground cumin*
*½ teaspoon cayenne pepper*
*14 scallops*

# Stuffed Shrimp

*Yields 4 servings*
Calories: 245
Fat: 8 grams
Protein: 30 grams
Carbohydrates: 13 grams
Cholesterol: 246 milligrams

*light cooking spray*
*1 pound cooked shrimp, peeled*
*1 tablespoon butter*
*½ onion, finely chopped*
*¼ cup celery, finely chopped*
*½ teaspoon lemon juice*
*½ cup cooked crabmeat*
*½ cup bread crumbs*
*1 egg, beaten*

You can buy prepackaged cooked crabmeat in the seafood section of your grocery store.

1. Preheat broiler. Prepare a baking sheet with light cooking spray.

2. Butterfly the shrimp and place on the baking sheet. Set aside.

3. Sauté chopped onions and celery in butter and lemon for 3 minutes.

4. Add crabmeat, breadcrumbs, and ½ of the beaten egg to onion and celery mixture and remove from heat, still mixing. Discard remaining egg.

5. Spoon equal amounts of breadcrumb mixture onto butterflied shrimp.

6. Broil for 6 minutes or until browned.

## Butterflying Shrimp

To butterfly a shrimp, split it down the back with a knife, cutting just enough to pull the sides apart but not enough to cut the shrimp in half. The shrimp opens like a butterfly with its wings unfurled. This cooking technique is used for other meats as well, including fish and poultry.

# Shrimp Scampi

Shrimp scampi is usually served with a melted butter mixture instead of vegetable oil. You can melt some butter or margarine instead of the oil, but be sure to factor in the calorie count of ¼ cup of melted butter.

1. Preheat oven to 350°F. Prepare a baking pan with light cooking spray.

2. In a medium bowl, mix the vegetable oil, lemon juice, garlic, parsley, and salt.

3. Add the shrimp to the mixture, tossing to coat.

4. Evenly distribute shrimp in the baking pan. Drizzle the mixture over the shrimp.

5. Bake for 5 minutes and turn shrimp. Bake another 5 minutes or until done.

6. Garnish with lemon slices or wedges before serving.

*Yields 4 servings*
Calories: 240
Fat: 16 grams
Protein: 25 grams
Carbohydrates: 3 grams
Cholesterol: 223 milligrams

*light cooking spray*
*¼ cup vegetable oil*
*1 tablespoon lemon juice*
*4 cloves garlic, crushed*
*¼ cup fresh parsley, chopped*
*1 teaspoon salt*
*1 pound cooked shrimp*
*1 lemon, sliced or wedged*

# Sautéed Shrimp

*Peel and devein your shrimp before you cook it. Leaving the tails on or removing them is purely a matter of personal preference.*

1. Heat the olive oil in a skillet over medium heat.

2. Add the crushed garlic and sauté for 3 minutes, gently mixing and tossing the garlic. Squeeze a lemon on the garlic as it sautés, gently mixing.

3. Add the shrimp and gently toss in the lemon, olive oil, and garlic mixture.

4. Squeeze more lemon into the sauté; continue tossing until shrimp is done, about 6 minutes.

### Deveining Shrimp
With a small, sharp paring knife, gently pull the vein out of the back of the shrimp. Use the knife to gently pierce the skin of the shrimp to tease the vein out, being careful not to cut yourself.

*Yields 4 servings*
Calories: 248
Fat: 16 grams
Protein: 23 grams
Carbohydrates: 3 grams
Cholesterol: 23 milligrams

¼ cup olive oil
3 cloves garlic, crushed
1 lemon
1 pound uncooked shrimp

# Mama's Gingered Shrimp

*The key to making this shrimp is the marinating. The longer you marinate, the better the taste.*

1. Mix the oil, soy sauce, and cider vinegar in a medium bowl. Add the ginger root, garlic, and scallion. Salt and pepper to taste.

2. Mix in the shrimp, tossing to coat evenly. Allow shrimp to marinate for 2 hours, tossing every 30 minutes.

3. Pour shrimp and marinade into a skillet and sauté over medium heat until cooked.

### Gingered Shrimp Salad
This recipe makes an unbelievably delicious salad. Toss the gingered shrimp in a bed of mixed greens. Add chopped tomatoes, hardboiled egg, and sunflower seeds, and you have a beautiful gingered shrimp salad.

*Yields 4 servings*
Calories: 253
Fat: 16 grams
Protein: 24 grams
Carbohydrates: 3 grams
Cholesterol: 173 milligrams

3 tablespoons low-sodium soy
    sauce
¼ cup vegetable oil
2 teaspoons cider vinegar
2" piece fresh ginger root, peeled
    and minced
1 clove garlic, minced
1 scallion, minced
salt and pepper to taste
1 pound uncooked shrimp, deveined
    and peeled

The Everything Calorie Counting Cookbook

# Sweet and Sour Shrimp

*You can add sliced onion and peppers to this if you want
to bulk it up without too many additional calories.*

1. Marinate the shrimp in soy sauce for 3–4 hours.

2. Separate the shrimp from the marinade and add in the rice wine vinegar, Splenda brown sugar, ginger, garlic, and the pineapple juice.

3. Heat olive oil in a wok over medium heat. Add the marinade and the shrimp and toss until the shrimp is cooked. Pour the shrimp and marinade back into the bowl and set aside.

4. Stir-fry the celery and carrot chunks until soft.

5. Add the pineapple chunks and the shrimp. Toss everything together for 2 minutes.

6. Remove wok from heat and pour over rice.

*Yields 4 servings*
Calories: 470
Fat: 18 grams
Protein: 49 grams
Carbohydrates: 29 grams
Cholesterol: 345 milligrams

*2 pounds shrimp, peeled and
    deveined*
*¼ cup soy sauce*
*2 tablespoons rice wine vinegar*
*2 tablespoons Splenda brown sugar*
*1 teaspoon ground ginger*
*1 clove garlic, crushed*
*1 10-ounce can pineapple chunks in
    juice*
*¼ cup olive oil*
*1 stalk celery, cut in chunks*
*1 carrot, cut in chunks*
*1½ cups rice*

# Shrimp with Angel Hair Pasta

**Yields 4 servings**
Calories: 475
Fat: 18 grams
Protein: 33 grams
Carbohydrates: 45 grams
Cholesterol: 176 milligrams

¼ cup olive oil
1 pound uncooked shrimp, deveined
    and peeled
1 lemon
½ pound angel hair pasta, cooked
¼ cup grated parmesan cheese

If you like spicy shrimp, add 1 teaspoon red pepper flakes to the shrimp sauté.

1. Heat oil in a skillet over medium heat. Add shrimp to skillet and sauté. Squeeze lemon over shrimp and toss shrimp until cooked. Drain oil from shrimp and pour over cooked pasta.

2. Toss the shrimp in the pasta and sprinkle with parmesan. Serve immediately.

### Quick Dinners

Sautéeing shrimp and cooking pasta is quick work. It should only take you about 15 minutes to prepare this meal. It's ideal for dinner parties when you want to spend your time with your guests, not your kitchen appliances. Garlic bread and a leafy green salad perfectly compliment this meal, and they're simple and fast to prepare, too!

# Shrimp and Chicken Jambalaya

*If you like chili powder, add it in with the chicken broth to your liking.*

1. Heat olive oil in a large skillet over medium heat. Add the onion, garlic, and peppers. Stir until the onions begin to soften, adding a spoonful or two of water if necessary to keep the mixture from sticking.

2. Stir in the tomatoes, chicken broth, thyme, basil, cayenne, cloves, and allspice. Bring to a boil, reduce heat, and simmer for 5 minutes.

3. Stir in the rice. Return to a boil, reduce heat, and cover.

4. Cook for 20 minutes, then add the shrimp, chicken, and parsley.

5. Simmer until the rice is done and the shrimp and chicken are cooked.

**_Yields 4 servings_**
Calories: 425
Fat: 8 grams
Protein: 45 grams
Carbohydrates: 44 grams
Cholesterol: 206 milligrams

1 tablespoon olive oil
1 onion, chopped
3 cloves garlic, minced
1 red pepper, chopped
1 green pepper, chopped
1 16-ounce can chopped tomatoes
    with juice
3 cups low-sodium chicken broth
1 teaspoon dried thyme
1 teaspoon dried basil
⅛ teaspoon cayenne pepper
⅛ teaspoon ground cloves
⅛ teaspoon ground allspice
¾ cups long grain rice
1 pound shrimp, deveined and
    peeled
2 chicken breast fillets, sliced in thin
    strips
2 tablespoons chopped fresh
    parsley

# Maryland Crab Cakes

Even store-bought crabmeat can sometimes have thin bones
in it, so be sure to pick it over thoroughly before you begin cooking.

**Yields 4 servings**
Calories: 165
Fat: 7 grams
Protein: 26 grams
Carbohydrates: 1.5 grams
Cholesterol: 134 milligrams

1 egg
1 teaspoon Old Bay seasoning
1 teaspoon light mayonnaise
salt and pepper to taste
1 teaspoon Worcestershire sauce
¼ cup fresh parsley, chopped
½ onion, finely chopped
1 pound lump crabmeat, cooked
1 tablespoon olive oil

1. Beat the egg in a medium bowl. Add the Old Bay seasoning, mayonnaise, salt, pepper, Worcestershire sauce, parsley, and onion. Add the crabmeat and mix together thoroughly. Make into cakes, about 2" in diameter.

2. Heat olive oil on medium in a large skillet. Add the crab cakes and cook until golden brown on both sides.

### Maryland Crabs

Maryland is renowned for its delicious native crabs. The Chesapeake Bay yields some of the world's tastiest crustaceans. Different areas around the bay vary in the way they prepare their crab cakes. This particular mayonnaise-based crab mix is more popular in urban areas. Other parts of the state delight in delicate crab cakes with crab, butter, and almost no additional ingredients.

# Spicy Crab Cakes

*This recipe makes six large crab cakes, about 4 inches wide.*

1. Mix bread crumbs and ½ of the parsley in a medium bowl. Set aside.

2. Pulse the egg, lemon juice, Worcestershire sauce, Tabasco sauce, paprika, and black pepper in a food processor. Between pulses, add the olive oil and mix on high until thickened. Transfer to a medium bowl and set aside.

3. In a large bowl, combine the onion, bell pepper, and the remaining parsley. Add the egg mixture and crab meat, blending slowly. Add half of the bread crumbs, working lightly so the crumbs stay crunchy.

4. Make 6 crab cakes and dredge them in the remaining bread crumbs.

5. In a large skillet add 2 tablespoons olive oil and fry the crab cakes until brown on each side.

*__Yields 6 servings__*
Calories: 348
Fat: 9 grams
Protein: 25 grams
Carbohydrates: 43 grams
Cholesterol: 88 milligrams

*3 cups bread crumbs*
*½ cup fresh chopped parsley, divided*
*1 egg*
*2 teaspoons lemon juice*
*2 teaspoons Worcestershire sauce*
*1 teaspoon Tabasco sauce*
*1 teaspoon paprika*
*½ teaspoon freshly ground black pepper*
*5 teaspoons olive oil*
*1 onion, chopped*
*¼ cup chopped green bell pepper*
*¼ cup chopped red bell pepper*
*1 pound lump crabmeat*

# Crab and Corn Pasta

**Yields 6 servings**
Calories: 307
Fat: 11 grams
Protein: 22 grams
Carbohydrates: 34 grams
Cholesterol: 53 milligrams

½ pound whole wheat pasta,
    cooked
½ cup whole kernel corn
¼ cup olive oil
1 lemon
1 pound lump crabmeat

What makes this recipe so unique is the crunch from the uncooked corn.
To make it really pop, use frozen corn so it's cold.

1.  Mix pasta, corn, olive oil, lemon juice, and crabmeat, tossing gently.

### Crabmeat

You can use nearly any type of crabmeat for this recipe, but blue crab and Dungeness are best because they are sweet to the taste. Dungeness crabs are found along the Pacific Coast of North America, and strict regulations prevent overtaxing the population. Similar measures are in place to protect blue crabs, but their populations are still on the decline.

# 12

# Chicken & Turkey

# Chicken Fajitas

*You can kick these up by adding jalapeño peppers.*

## Yields 4 servings
Calories: 240
Fat: 9 grams
Protein: 28 grams
Carbohydrates: 12 grams
Cholesterol: 66 milligrams

*1 pound skinless, boneless chicken breasts*
*2 tablespoons canola oil*
*1 red or green pepper thinly sliced and de-seeded*
*1 small Vidalia onion, thinly sliced lengthwise*
*1 cup unsalted mild or medium salsa*
*4 large wonton wrappers or 4 corn or flour tortillas*
*salt and pepper to taste*

1. Heat canola oil in frying pan and fry chicken breasts on both sides.

2. Cut fried chicken into long 1" strips.

3. Stir-fry green pepper strips and onion strips in canola oil until tender.

4. Combine peppers, onions, and salsa. Pour over chicken strips.

5. Spoon chicken mix into warm tortillas or wonton wraps.

## Warming Tortillas

Serve the fajita mixture on warm tortillas by heating the tortillas for 10–15 seconds in the microwave or for 2 minutes in a 200°F oven. You can leave them in a little longer if you want them crispier. This is a great low-calorie solution for high-fat frying your tortillas.

# Chicken Salad

You can cook the chicken breasts a variety of ways, including boiling, baking, or even frying. You can also purchase cooked chicken strips and chop them up for this salad.

1. Mix ingredients together and chill.

2. Serve on a bed of lettuce.

### Chicken Salad: A Classic

Chicken salad is one of America's most popular dishes because it is light and easy to make. It's a great way to use up leftover chicken, and it's a surefire favorite at gatherings. Just be careful to keep it refrigerated as much as possible; mayonnaise and warmth don't go together well.

**_Yields 4 servings_**
Calories: 263
Fat: 7 grams
Protein: 34 grams
Carbohydrates: 15 grams
Cholesterol: 191 milligrams

3 cups cooked chicken breasts, chopped
1 cup celery, chopped
⅓ cup pickle relish
2 hard boiled eggs, chopped
¾ cup fat-free mayonnaise
4 lettuce leaves

# Baked Chicken

_Yields 4 servings_
Calories: 230
Fat: 7 grams
Protein: 33 grams
Carbohydrates: 8 grams
Cholesterol: 80 milligrams

light cooking spray
4 4-ounce boneless, skinless chicken
    breasts
salt and pepper to taste
1 10-ounce can cream of chicken
    soup
½ cup low-fat shredded Swiss
    cheese

You can replace the cream of chicken soup with low sodium chicken broth if you prefer.

1. Preheat oven to 350°F.

2. Spray baking pan with light cooking spray.

3. Arrange chicken in pan. Sprinkle salt and pepper on both sides to taste.

4. Pour in chicken soup and one can of water.

5. Cover with foil and bake for 30 minutes.

6. Uncover chicken and sprinkle with Swiss cheese.

7. Bake for an extra 15 minutes.

## Go Nuts!

Crush pecans and sprinkle them over the chicken alone or with the shredded cheese for an extra crunch. Try more exotic nuts in your poultry dishes. Gingko nuts, the fruit of the gingko biloba, are preserved in brine and sold at specialty stores. They make a soft, sweet addition to poultry dishes.

# Sweet and Sour Chicken

*This is a simple sweet and sour chicken recipe that you can
throw together at the last minute for dinner guests.*

1. Preheat oven to 350°F.

2. Heat canola oil in a skillet. Brown chicken breasts.

3. Transfer chicken to a baking dish.

4. Combine onion soup mix, orange juice, and water in small bowl and pour
   over the chicken.

5. Bake uncovered for 50 minutes.

*Yields 4 servings*
Calories: 295
Fat: 9 grams
Protein: 29 grams
Carbohydrates: 25 grams
Cholesterol: 69 grams

*2 tablespoons canola oil*
*4 4-ounce boneless, skinless chicken*
   *breasts*
*1 package dry onion soup mix*
*1 6-ounce can frozen orange juice*
   *concentrate, thawed*
*½ cup water*

# Balsamic Chicken and Mushrooms

*Yields 6 servings*
Calories: 187
Fat: 6 grams
Protein: 11 grams
Carbohydrates: 23 grams
Cholesterol: 21 milligrams

*light olive oil cooking spray*
*1 16-ounce package frozen onions*
*and peppers*
*1 8-ounce package sliced*
*mushrooms*
*1 tablespoon balsamic vinegar*
*¾ can cream of mushroom soup*
*diluted in ¾ can water*
*1 cup nonfat milk*
*5-pound roasted chicken, cut into*
*pieces*
*minced garlic to taste*
*2 cups rice, cooked*

*Olive oil spray is recommended with this recipe because it*
*adds to the overall taste of the chicken and mushrooms.*

1. Spray a large skillet with olive oil spray.

2. Cook the pepper and onions with the mushrooms until the onions are translucent.

3. Stir in balsamic vinegar.

4. Stir in mushroom soup, milk, roasted chicken, and garlic.

5. Boil for 1 minute, then reduce heat and simmer for 10 minutes.

6. Serve over cooked rice.

## Roasting Chicken

You can purchase a pre-roasted chicken for this recipe or you can roast one yourself. Rinse a whole chicken and dry it with paper towels. Salt and pepper the bird inside and out; this will create the crisp, salty flavor a roasted chicken should have. Bake in the oven at 425°F for 1 hour.

# Chicken and Green Bean Casserole

*You can replace Italian bread crumbs with croutons. Simply pour a bag of croutons into a resealable plastic bag and mash them up to make crumbs.*

1. Preheat oven to 350°F.

2. Combine soup, soy sauce, and pepper in a medium bowl. Stir in beans.

3. Place chicken in a baking dish. Sprinkle salt and pepper over to taste.

4. Cover chicken with the bean mixture. Sprinkle with bread crumbs.

5. Bake for 20 minutes.

*Yields 4 servings*
Calories: 318
Fat: 7 grams
Protein: 32 grams
Carbohydrates: 30 grams
Cholesterol: 69 milligrams

*1 10-ounce can cream of mushroom soup, diluted in 1 can water*
*1 teaspoon low-sodium soy sauce*
*pepper to taste*
*1 9-ounce box frozen cut green beans, thawed*
*1 pound chicken breasts, cooked and sliced*
*1 cup Italian bread crumbs*

# Chicken and Dumplings

A store-bought roasted chicken is fine for this recipe or you can prepare it yourself. Baked chicken is another tasty alternative.

_Yields 8 servings_
Calories: 683
Fat: 39 grams
Protein: 59 grams
Carbohydrates: 23 grams
Cholesterol: 175 milligrams

4 pounds whole roasted chicken
2 tablespoons canola oil
1 large onion, chopped
3 large stalks celery, chopped
3 large carrots, chopped
1 tablespoon poultry seasoning
16 ounces low-sodium chicken broth
1 10-ounce package buttermilk biscuits
1 9-ounce can low-fat chicken gravy

1. Shred chicken, removing skin and bones.

2. Heat canola oil in a skillet. Sauté the vegetables in the oil.

3. Place chicken, vegetables, and poultry seasoning into large pot. Add the chicken broth.

4. Bring to a boil. Reduce heat and simmer for 10 minutes.

5. Place biscuits one at a time into the chicken mix. Cover the pot and cook for 10 minutes.

6. Stir in chicken gravy. Simmer for several minutes and serve.

## Serving Dumplings

Chicken with dumplings is a popular Southern dish. If you prefer your biscuits crispier, you can wait to add them until after you pour the gravy in, about 5 minutes before you serve the dish.

The Everything Calorie Counting Cookbook

# Pulled Chicken

This is a simple pulled chicken recipe. The key is to make sure your chicken is soft and pulls apart very easily, just like pork.

1. Boil chicken breasts until tender.

2. Cool chicken and shred.

3. Stir chicken into bread crumbs.

4. Spread over hamburger buns and serve.

Calories: 312
Fat: 4 grams
Protein: 33 grams
Carbohydrates: 37 grams
Cholesterol: 66 milligrams

*6 4-ounce boneless, skinless chicken breasts*
*1 5.5-ounce package of plain bread crumbs*
*6 low-carb hamburger buns*

# Lemon Chicken

You can serve this over rice or with steamed vegetables. You might also want to add some chopped onions or garlic to this recipe.

**_Yields 4 servings_**
Calories: 150
Fat: 2 grams
Protein: 28 grams
Carbohydrates: 6 grams
Cholesterol: 69 milligrams

_4 4-ounce chicken breasts, skinned and boned_
_1 cup lemon juice_
_1 teaspoon lemon-pepper_
_2 tablespoons low-sodium soy sauce_

1. Marinate chicken breasts in lemon juice for 1 hour.

2. Preheat oven to 350°F.

3. Place chicken in baking dish.

4. Add soy sauce and lemon pepper on top of chicken.

5. Bake for 30 minutes.

## Marinating Tips

It is best to marinate in a non-reactive container, like glass. There are specially designed plastic containers for marinating meat, but a resealable plastic bag works just as well. Both options allow you to coat both sides of the meat without worrying about spilling the marinade.

The Everything Calorie Counting Cookbook

# No-Chunk Crunchy Baked Chicken

*The best way to bake chicken is to arrange the breasts in a
single layer, not touching, in a greased shallow baking dish.*

1. Preheat oven to 350°F.

2. Combine the bread crumbs and Parmesan in a medium bowl.

3. Salt and pepper to taste.

4. Dip chicken breasts in melted butter, then coat with the bread crumb mixture.

5. Spray chicken with butter-flavored cooking spray.

6. Place chicken in baking dish and cover with aluminum foil.

7. Bake for 30 minutes or until tender.

*Yields 4 servings*
Calories: 328
Fat: 16 grams
Protein: 33 grams
Carbohydrates: 10 grams
Cholesterol: 78 milligrams

*½ cup dry bread crumbs*
*½ cup Parmesan cheese*
*salt and pepper to taste*
*¼ cup melted margarine*
*4 4-ounce skinless, boneless chicken
    breasts*
*butter-flavored cooking spray*

# Broiled Herb Chicken

*Yields 4 servings*
Calories: 303
Fat: 18 grams
Protein: 28 grams
Carbohydrates: 7 grams
Cholesterol: 69 milligrams

*4 4-ounce boneless, skinless chicken
  breasts*
*1 8-ounce bottle Italian salad
  dressing*
*2 tablespoons parsley flakes*

*When you marinate meats, you need to flip them in the
marinade several times to be sure to soak all sides.*

1. Marinate chicken breasts in Italian dressing for 1 hour.

2. Place marinated chicken on a grilling pan and sprinkle with parsley flakes.

3. Broil chicken breasts on both sides until done.

## Broiling Tips

To make sure your broiler is hot enough, start by heating your oven to its maximum temperature and then turn on the broiler. While the oven is preheating, leave a cast-iron or heavy-duty steel skillet inside so it's hot as well when you start broiling the chicken breasts.

# Oven-Fried Chicken

*Be sure to crush corn flakes thoroughly. This makes the fried chicken so crispy you won't even remember you used corn flakes.*

1. Mix sour cream with the salad dressing in a small bowl.

2. Place chicken breasts in a plastic bag and add the sour cream and Italian salad dressing. Mix and refrigerate for 1 hour.

3. Preheat oven to 375°F.

4. Remove chicken and shake off excess liquid

5. Dredge chicken in crushed corn flakes.

6. Place in baking dish and bake for 45 minutes.

*Yields 2 servings;*
*serving size 4 ounces*
Calories: 255
Fat: 4 grams
Protein: 31 grams
Carbohydrates: 25 grams
Cholesterol: 73 milligrams

*¼ cup fat-free sour cream*
*¼ cup low-calorie Italian salad*
*    dressing*
*2 4-ounce skinless, boneless chicken*
*    breasts*
*1½ cups crushed corn flakes*

# Vancho Chicken Paprikas

If you like mustard, add ¼ cup to the mixture.

Calories: 238
Fat: 6 grams
Protein: 30 grams
Carbohydrates: 14 grams
Cholesterol: 76 milligrams

1 10-ounce can cream of chicken
    soup
1 8-ounce carton fat-free sour
    cream
2 tablespoons Hungarian sweet
    paprika
4 4-ounce boneless, skinless chicken
    breasts

1. Preheat oven to 375°F.

2. Combine soup, sour cream, and paprika in a medium bowl.

3. Place chicken in a baking dish and cover chicken with mixture.

4. Bake for 1 hour.

## Hungarian Paprika

Hungary is known for its sweet, spicy paprika, and this is a regular dish in any good Hungarian home. It is traditionally served with potato dumplings, pickled Hungarian peppers, and lots of thick and crusty home-baked bread.

# Chicken Paella

This is truly a very simple dish because you can add or delete just about anything you like to the sauté and still have perfect paella. You might like to overcook the rice a little until it's crispy, which is how it is traditionally served.

1. Place chicken and shrimp in a plastic bag. Add Creole seasoning and shake to coat.

2. Heat canola oil in a pan. Add the chicken and sauté for about 10 minutes.

3. Add cod and shrimp and sauté for 2 minutes.

4. Add chicken stock, chorizo, wine, garlic, onion, salt, pepper, and clams and let stand over low heat until chicken is fully cooked.

5. Add green peas and cooked yellow rice. Cook until the rice absorbs all the chicken stock.

6. Place on a platter and garnish with cilantro leaves.

## Paella

Paella originated in Spain and is traditionally eaten on Sundays. It is usually served with vegetables, meat, or seafood. The main ingredients are always rice, saffron, and olive oil. You can try any combination of seafood or omit all meats and add more vegetables for a vegetarian-friendly option.

*Yields 4 servings*
Calories: 504
Fat: 27 grams
Protein: 36 grams
Carbohydrates: 26 grams
Cholesterol: 123 milligrams

½ pound chicken tenders, cut up
½ pound large, raw shrimp
4 teaspoons Creole seasoning
¼ cup canola oil
½ pound cod fillets
1 medium onion, quartered
2 cloves garlic, chopped
2 cups chicken stock
1 pound sliced chorizo sausage, cut into small pieces
½ cup white wine
salt and pepper to taste
1 pound clams
1 cup frozen peas
2 cups yellow rice, cooked
cilantro leaves, for garnish

# Chicken Marsala

Many people like to flatten their chicken before cooking. You can do this by placing the chicken breasts between two pieces of wax paper and pounding them with a meat pounder until thin. If you don't have a meat pounder, use the side of a skillet. Just make sure you pound all breasts to equal thickness or they will not cook evenly.

1. Mix salt and pepper in flour.

2. Dredge chicken breasts in flour.

3. Heat canola oil in large pan.

4. Fry chicken on both sides until brown, about 5 minutes for each side.

5. Remove chicken from pan. Add ham to the skillet to sauté for 1 minute.

6. Take out ham and sauté mushrooms until they are brown and dry.

7. Pour Marsala wine into the pan to boil down, about 10 seconds.

8. Add chicken stock and simmer for a minute.

9. Stir in butter and add chicken.

10. Simmer until chicken is heated through.

11. Season to taste and garnish with parsley before serving.

_**Yields 4 servings**_
Calories: 748
Fat: 52 grams
Protein: 35 grams
Carbohydrates: 30 grams
Cholesterol: 94 milligrams

*1 cup flour*
*salt and pepper to taste*
*4 4-ounce skinless, boneless chicken breasts*
*¼ cup canola oil*
*3–4 slices prosciutto ham, thinly sliced*
*½ cup sliced porcini mushrooms*
*½ cup sweet Marsala wine*
*½ cup chicken stock*
*2 tablespoons unsalted butter*
*½ cup flat-leaf parsley*

# Roast Chicken and Vegetables

Salting the cavity of the chicken will season the meat more effectively. Coat the inside with salt using your fingers or a cloth. You can also stuff this area with herbs, garlic, lemon wedges, and onions to perfume the meat.

1. Preheat oven to 375°F.

2. Combine all ingredients except chicken in a roasting pan.

3. Place chicken on top of mixture and add salt all over body to taste.

4. Bake uncovered for 1 hour.

## Trussing Chicken

Trussing helps the chicken keep its shape and cook more evenly during roasting. The easiest way is to simply tie the legs together with kitchen twine. The same goes for other birds such as turkey. Kitchen twine also comes in handy for tying herb bundles and performing other simple kitchen tasks.

*Yields 4 servings*
Calories: 873
Fat: 59 grams
Protein: 62 grams
Carbohydrates: 21 grams
Cholesterol: 251 milligrams

1 10-ounce can cream of mushroom
    soup
2 teaspoons crushed oregano leaves
1 16-ounce bag mixed vegetables
1 3-pound chicken
salt and pepper to taste

# Cornish Hen with Orange Glaze

*Pineapple makes a yummy glaze for these birds, too. Mix the juice from
a can of chopped pineapple with the butter and pour over hens.*

**Yields 6 servings**
Calories: 177
Fat: 10 grams
Protein: 5 grams
Carbohydrates: 17 grams
Cholesterol: 43 milligrams

*4 1½-pound Cornish hens, washed
    and dried*
*3 tablespoons butter, melted*
*1 10-ounce jar low-sugar orange
    marmalade*

1. Preheat oven to 350°F.

2. Bake hens for 30 minutes.

3. Melt the butter and marmalade in a microwave for 10 seconds.

4. Pour marmalade mixture over hens and bake for another hour, basting
   several times.

## Cornish Hens

Cornish hens are small chickens. They are actually a cross between a Cornish chicken and
another breed called the White Rock. Their petite size translates into the perfect serving
size. They yield all white meat, and their tender meat falls off the bone when they are prepared
correctly.

# Turkey Jambalaya

*Substitute steamed mussels or clams for the turkey to get a seafood jambalaya.*

1. In a large pan, combine stewed tomatoes, soup mix, and red pepper in two cups of water.

2. Bring to a boil, stirring well.

3. Reduce heat. Cover and simmer for 15 minutes.

4. Stir in turkey and ham. Simmer for 5 more minutes.

5. Pour over hot cooked rice.

### Jambalaya

Jambalaya is traditionally made by combining all ingredients in one pot and completed by adding rice. Generally, it's a very spicy dish, but you can regulate the heat in your own cooking by adding more or less crushed red pepper. You can also experiment with the vegetables in this dish depending on what you like and what's in season.

**Yields 4 servings**
Calories: 363
Fat: 7 grams
Protein: 43 grams
Carbohydrates: 31 grams
Cholesterol: 100 milligrams

1 15-ounce can stewed tomatoes
1 package dry vegetable soup mix
1 teaspoon crushed red pepper
1 cup low-fat ham, cut into thin strips
2 cups cooked turkey, chopped
2 cups cooked basmati rice

# John's Turkey Chili

**_Yields 4 servings_**
Calories: 590
Fat: 32 grams
Protein: 62 grams
Carbohydrates: 15 grams
Cholesterol: 186 milligrams

2 pounds ground turkey
⅓ teaspoon garlic powder
chili powder to taste
1 teaspoon Splenda
1 8-ounce can tomato sauce
2 cups shredded Monterey jack
    cheese
1 cup fat-free sour cream

Serve this turkey chili recipe with tortilla chips. You can even use the tortilla chips as a base, placing them in the bottom of the bowl and pouring the chili on top to serve. This chili tastes even better the next day after the juices have soaked into the meat.

1. Combine turkey and garlic powder with ½ cup water in a large saucepan. Cook over medium heat for 5–6 min.

2. Add chili powder, Splenda, and tomato sauce and simmer until meat is tender.

3. Serve in bowls and garnish with fat-free sour cream or cheese.

### The Multitalented Turkey

Turkey is a healthy, lean meat that is packed with protein and contains vitamin B6, which helps your body produce energy. These days it is easy to incorporate turkey into your diet because you can buy turkey cutlets, ground turkey, and turkey breasts instead of just a whole turkey.

# Turkey Casserole

This casserole tastes good served over whole wheat noodles or cooked rice.

1. Preheat oven to 350°F.

2. Mix all ingredients together in a large bowl.

3. Place ingredients in a lightly sprayed cooking dish.

4. Bake uncovered for 35 minutes.

## Casseroles

Casseroles date back to the early 18th century when meat was slowly cooked in clay containers with rice. Today you can bake them in the oven and they can be ready in less than an hour. You can also adapt your recipe for an easy slow-cooker meal.

*Yields 4 servings*
Calories: 498
Fat: 9 grams
Protein: 36 grams
Carbohydrates: 69 grams
Cholesterol: 78 milligrams

3 cups cooked light meat turkey
1 8-ounce can pineapple chunks, drained
½ cup apricot preserves
1 10-ounce can cream of chicken soup
1 8-ounce can sliced water chestnuts
⅓ cup water
2 cups cooked rice
light cooking spray

# John's Turkey Tacos

*You can incorporate chopped tomatoes to add flavor and bulk to these delicious tortillas.*

**Yields 4 servings**
Calories: 553
Fat: 28 grams
Protein: 23 grams
Carbohydrates: 51 grams
Cholesterol: 43 milligrams

*2 tablespoons canola oil*
*½ pound lean ground turkey*
*1 small onion, diced*
*1 16-ounce jar mild salsa*
*½ cup shredded low-fat Mexican-*
*    blend cheese*
*1 ripe avocado*
*8 soft flour tortillas*
*salt and pepper to taste*
*6 iceberg lettuce leaves, shredded*

1. Cook turkey meat in canola oil until brown over medium heat in a medium cooking pot.

2. In a sauté pan, sauté onion until translucent. Combine onion with salsa and ½ cup water in a small bowl. Add meat to onion and salsa mixture. Add the cheese and stir.

3. Remove skin from avocado. Smash avocado in another bowl and season to taste.

4. Wrap tortillas in moist paper towels. Heat tortillas in microwave for 1 minute. Flatten tortillas and divide turkey mixture evenly on top. Top with avocado and lettuce. Fold over and serve with extra shredded cheese and salsa.

# Turkey Salad

**Yields 4 servings**
Calories 440
Fat: 23 grams
Protein: 35 grams
Carbohydrates: 27 grams
Cholesterol: 85 milligrams

*3 cups chopped cooked turkey*
*1 cup chopped celery*
*1 cup chopped granny apple*
*1 10-ounce can mandarin oranges,*
*    drained*
*½ cup chopped macadamia nuts*
*1 teaspoon curry powder*
*¾ cup fat-free mayonnaise*
*6 large lettuce leaves*

*Cook turkey in a medium cooking pot on medium heat, stirring as you go. It is best when served a little warm with this salad.*

1. Mix turkey with celery, apple, oranges, and nuts. Add curry powder and mayonnaise.

2. Serve on lettuce leaves.

# 13

# Vegetarian

# Grilled Artichokes

*When grilling artichoke leaves, use a vegetable grilling pan
with holes so you don't lose the leaves into the grill.*

**Yields 6 servings**
Calories: 137
Fat: 9 grams
Protein: 3 grams
Carbohydrates: 14 grams
Cholesterol: 0 milligrams

*3 large artichokes*
*4 cups water*
*1 lemon*
*¼ cup olive oil*
*3 tablespoons Worcestershire sauce*
*1 tablespoon honey*
*1 clove garlic, minced*

1. Boil artichokes until tender; the leaves should pull out easily. Remove the artichokes from the water and pull the leaves out.

2. Squeeze the juice of one lemon into a medium bowl. Add the olive oil, Worcestershire sauce, honey, and garlic. Mix ingredients well; dip the leaves in the mixture.

3. Turn grill on to medium heat. Add artichoke leaves to grilling pan and grill until slightly charred around edges.

4. Sprinkle with salt and pepper to taste. Serve hot.

# Crunchy Eggplant

*These can be served hot or cold. Served cold they taste like eggplant potato chips.*

1. Preheat oven to 350°F.

2. Mix egg whites, salt, pepper, paprika, and garlic in a small bowl.

3. Dredge eggplant slices through this mixture, coating evenly on all sides.

4. Place slices on baking sheet. Sprinkle with parmesan cheese. Bake for 30 minutes or until crispy.

## Eggplant

The Latin name for eggplant is "mad apple." There was a time when Europeans believed that the eggplant caused you to go insane if you ate it. It was Thomas Jefferson who introduced the eggplant to the United States after he took a trip to France and fell in love with the taste.

*Yields 3 servings*
Calories: 97
Fat: 2 grams
Protein: 8 grams
Carbohydrates: 12 grams
Cholesterol: 7 milligrams

*3 egg whites, whipped*
*1 teaspoon salt*
*1 teaspoon pepper*
*1 teaspoon paprika*
*1 clove garlic, minced*
*1 eggplant, sliced*
*4 tablespoons Parmesan cheese*

# Sweet Potato Puff

**Yields 8 servings**
Calories: 145
Fat: 6 grams
Protein: 4 grams
Carbohydrates: 21 grams
Cholesterol: 0 milligrams

light cooking spray
3 cups cooked sweet potatoes,
    chopped into little cubes
4 egg whites
¼ cup Splenda
1 teaspoon vanilla
½ cup orange juice
2 tablespoons flour
1 teaspoon salt
½ cup chopped pecans

This is a Southern specialty that usually involves a lot of sugar, but this recipe substitutes Splenda. You can use virtually any nut to top it, but pecans work well with the sweet flavors.

1. Preheat oven to 350°F. Lightly spray a casserole or baking dish.

2. Place all ingredients in a blender or food processor and puree. Transfer to a baking dish. Sprinkle chopped pecans on top. Bake about 30 minutes and serve.

## Serving Sweet Potato Puffs

To serve, use an ice cream scoop to scoop out each puff so it's a nice, puffy ball on your plate. You can also top with more sprinkled pecans, and it's also great served atop a bed of green beans.

# Baked French Fries

*The grated parmesan really snaps these fries up. You can also add black pepper and chili powder if you like them spicy.*

1. Preheat oven to 450°F.

2. Cut the potatoes into wedges.

3. In a small bowl, mix the olive oil, paprika, garlic powder, onion powder, and parmesan.

4. Dip each wedge in the mixture to coat evenly.

5. Place wedges on a baking sheet, bake about 40 minutes or until golden brown.

**_Yields 2 servings_**
Calories: 420
Fat: 15 grams
Protein: 9 grams
Carbohydrates: 67 grams
Cholesterol: 3 milligrams

*2 large Idaho potatoes*
*2 tablespoons olive oil*
*1 teaspoon paprika*
*1 teaspoon garlic powder*
*1 teaspoon onion powder*
*2 teaspoons grated Parmesan cheese*

# Vegetable Stuffed Peppers

**Yields 4 servings**
Calories: 278
Fat: 6 grams
Protein: 14 grams
Carbohydrates: 41 grams
Cholesterol: 5 milligrams

4 green bell peppers
6 cups water
1 15-ounce can pinto beans, rinsed
    and drained
2 cups whole kernel corn
¾ cup low-fat shredded cheddar cheese
½ tablespoon vegetable oil
1 clove garlic, crushed
½ onion, chopped
1 teaspoon black pepper

When you place the peppers on the baking pan, add a little water to the pan so that the peppers don't burn.

1. Preheat oven to 375°F.

2. Cut off the tops of the green peppers. Remove the seeds.

3. Boil six cups of water; add peppers and cook for 5 minutes. Remove peppers, place upside down on a paper towel to drain.

4. Mix all remaining ingredients in a medium bowl. Divide ingredients evenly among peppers and stuff them. Place peppers on a baking dish, filled side up, bake about 20 minutes. Serve hot.

# Jalapeño Tortilla Roll-Ups

*You can get very creative with this recipe and add
anything you might want to roll up with the jalapeños.*

1. Cream the nonfat cream cheese in a medium bowl. Mix in the jalapeños, scallions, and garlic.

2. Add the salt, chili powder, and paprika. Evenly spread the mixture onto tortillas. Roll up the tortillas and wrap individually in clear plastic wrap.

3. Refrigerate for a few hours until cold; slice and serve.

*Yields 6 servings*
Calories: 208
Fat: 5 grams
Protein: 10 grams
Carbohydrates: 31 grams
Cholesterol: 3 milligrams

*1 cup nonfat cream cheese*
*1 8-ounce can chopped jalapeños*
*4 scallions, chopped*
*1 clove garlic, minced*
*1 teaspoon salt*
*1 teaspoon chili powder*
*1 teaspoon paprika*
*6 flour tortillas*

# Chickpea Quiche

**Yields 6 servings**
Calories: 455
Fat: 22 grams
Protein: 12 grams
Carbohydrates: 52 grams
Cholesterol: 3 milligrams

1 9" frozen pie shell
1 15-ounce can chickpeas
3 egg whites, well beaten
½ cup skim milk
2 tablespoons flour
½ cup chopped onion
½ cup shredded low-fat cheddar
    cheese

*Add more flour if you need to thicken the mix; add more skim milk if it's too thick.
The mixture should be fluid enough to pour into the pie crust but not watery.*

1. Preheat oven to 400°F.

2. Bake the pie shell for 7 minutes, remove from heat, and turn the oven down to 350°F.

3. Puree the chickpeas, egg whites, and skim milk in a blender. Add in the flour if the mix is too watery. Move mixture to a medium bowl, and add the onion.

4. Pour into the partially baked pie shell. Sprinkle the cheese over the top evenly. Bake for 35 minutes.

# Veggie-Stuffed Zucchini

*Stuff the zucchini with any vegetables you like. The vegetables
in this recipe can easily be substituted with your favorites.*

1. Preheat oven to 375°F.

2. Cut each zucchini in half lengthwise and scoop out the pulp. Place each half with the open side up on a shallow roasting pan and sprinkle with salt.

3. Heat margarine and oil in a skillet over medium heat. Add onion and garlic; sauté for 4 minutes, then stir in flour, coriander, potato, peas, and cilantro.

4. Spoon ¼ of potato mixture into each zucchini half and cover with foil.

5. Bake for 15 minutes or until zucchini is tender.

*Yields 4 servings*
Calories: 205
Fat: 5 grams
Protein: 8 grams
Carbohydrates: 35 grams
Cholesterol: 0 milligrams

*4 medium zucchini*
*1 teaspoon salt, divided four ways*
*2 teaspoons margarine*
*2 teaspoons vegetable oil*
*1 onion, chopped*
*1 clove garlic, crushed*
*½ cup chickpeas*
*2 tablespoons flour*
*1 teaspoon ground coriander*
*1 potato, peeled, cooked, and diced*
*1 cup green peas*
*2 tablespoons chopped cilantro*

# Polenta Pie

*Yields 8 servings*
Calories: 200
Fat: 4 grams
Protein: 6 grams
Carbohydrates: 39 grams
Cholesterol: 0 milligrams

5 teaspoons olive oil
1 onion, finely chopped
2 10-ounce packages chopped
    spinach
4 cloves garlic, crushed
salt and pepper to taste
3 cups water
3 cups low-sodium vegetable broth
2 cups coarse-ground yellow
    cornmeal
2 cups tomato sauce, any type
basil leaves to garnish

Microwave the tomato sauce to warm it before topping on slices of the polenta pie.

1. Preheat oven to 375°F. Lightly oil a ceramic quiche dish, set aside.

2. Heat 2 tablespoons of oil in a large skillet. Add the onion and sauté for about 2 minutes. Add the thawed spinach, sauté until soft. Add the garlic, salt, and pepper; continue to stir for 5 minutes, then set aside.

3. Combine the water, broth, and cornmeal in a medium bowl.

4. Spoon half of the polenta into the pie dish, pressing it down with your fingers or the back of a spoon to make a smooth surface. Spoon in the spinach filling, spreading evenly. Spoon in remaining polenta over spinach, spreading evenly. Brush top of polenta layer with remaining oil.

5. Cover with foil and bake for 30 minutes, then remove the foil and bake for another 15 minutes or until top is browned. Remove from oven, top each wedge with tomato sauce, and serve while hot.

## Polenta Possibilities

Polenta is ground, dried, white or yellow corn meal and was traditionally peasant food that now commands high prices. Using less water, you can make polenta like cornbread and grill it, or you can add more water to make thinner polenta that you can serve with sauce, meat, or cheese and treat like pasta.

# Vegetable Chowder

This is what you make when it's cold outside and you don't
want to run to the store. It's easy, filling, and delicious.

1. Melt margarine in a large, deep skillet over medium heat. Add the vegetables until tender, tossing occasionally. Add the water, broth, and potatoes; boil for 15 minutes or until potatoes are tender.

2. Add the milk, stirring to combine, and turn heat down to medium high. Add the flour to thicken. If you need to thicken further, add more flour. Serve hot.

## Buying Garlic

When buying fresh garlic, look for heads that are plump, firm, and heavy for their size. Any green shoots or sprouts indicate that the garlic is old and will have an off flavor. Store whole bulbs in an open plastic bag in the vegetable drawer of your refrigerator. Markets carry a variety of processed garlic options, but buy these in the smallest containers possible, since they lose their fresh taste and become stale very quickly.

*Yields 8 servings*
Calories: 158
Fat: 5 grams
Protein: 8 grams
Carbohydrates: 24 grams
Cholesterol: 2 milligrams

3 tablespoons margarine
1 onion, chopped
1 cup chopped celery
2 cups sliced carrots
½ cup water
3 cups low-sodium chicken or
    vegetable broth
3 potatoes, peeled and diced
3 cups skim milk
¼ cup flour

# Hearty Vegetable Stew

*To sweeten this stew, add 2 tablespoons of honey or Splenda.*
*This stew is great over rice, couscous or any other grain.*

*Yields 6 servings*
Calories: 347
Fat: 11 grams
Protein: 13 grams
Carbohydrates: 55 grams
Cholesterol: 0 milligrams

¼ cup olive oil
3 onions, chopped
4 carrots, chopped
2 red peppers, chopped
2 green peppers, chopped
4 stalks celery, chopped
1 cup mushrooms, halved
1 zucchini, sliced
1 14.5-ounce can green beans
1 14.5-ounce can peas
1 cup low-sodium tomato paste
salt to taste
2 tomatoes, chopped
1 15-ounce can chickpeas
1 cup water

1. Heat the olive oil in a deep skillet over medium heat. Sauté the vegetables. Add the tomato paste, a dash of salt, chickpeas and tomato slices. Add 1 cup of water and cook for 20 minutes over medium-high heat.

## Read the Label

The shelf life for a really good extra virgin olive oil is about two years. The label tells you a minimum of one important distinction: Extra Virgin. The International Olive Oil Commission (IOOC) has established that name to indicate that the oil was cold pressed, and that no chemicals were introduced to aid in extraction. It also indicates an acidity of less than 1 percent, which cannot be detected by taste. Oil must be analyzed in a laboratory to ascertain acidity level.

# Vegetarian Chili

You can serve this over rice, but it's also great served with large pieces
of lettuce, wrapped up like a taco and covered with hot sauce or
salsa if you prefer to keep it mild. It becomes a chili wrap!

1. Heat the olive oil in a deep skillet over medium heat. Add the onion, peppers, and garlic, and sauté for 15 minutes. Add the mushroom halves, beer and chili powder; mix well.

2. Turn heat up to high and add the tomatoes and beans; continue mixing.

3. Add in the ½ cup of vegetable stock and the cabbage; continue mixing.

4. Serve hot and squeeze lemon and lime over liberally to taste.

**_Yields 4 servings_**
Calories: 308
Fat: 9 grams
Protein: 13 grams
Carbohydrates: 54 grams
Cholesterol: 0 milligrams

2 tablespoons olive oil
2 onions, chopped finely
1 green pepper, chopped
1 red pepper, chopped
2 cloves garlic, minced
1 cup mushrooms, halved
½ cup beer
1 tablespoon chili powder
1 14-ounce can diced tomatoes
1 15-ounce can black beans, rinsed
   and drained
1 15-ounce can kidney beans, rinsed
   and drained
½ cup vegetable stock
1 cup shredded cabbage
1 lemon
1 lime

# Skinny Scalloped Potatoes

**Yields 8 servings**
Calories: 139
Fat: 5 grams
Protein: 8 grams
Carbohydrates: 19 grams
Cholesterol: 4 milligrams

*light cooking spray*
*4 Russet potatoes, peeled and thinly sliced*
*salt and pepper to taste*
*1 large onion, thinly sliced*
*½ cup nonfat cottage cheese*
*4 tablespoons chopped parsley*
*2 tablespoons chopped chives*
*3 tablespoons margarine*
*½ cup low-fat grated Swiss cheese*
*2 cups skim milk*

A 9" x 13" casserole dish is ideal, but if your dish is larger, keep in mind that the potatoes will cook faster because the ingredients are spread more thinly.

1. Preheat oven to 350°F. Lightly spray a casserole dish.

2. Layer bottom of dish with very thin potato slices. Sprinkle with salt and pepper.

3. Layer thin slices of onion over potato slices, then add the cottage cheese, 2 tablespoons of parsley, and 1 tablespoon of chives. Spread the margarine pieces over this layer.

4. Layer more potato slices and repeat as above using the Swiss cheese. Pour milk over the top layer.

5. Cover with aluminum foil and bake for one hour, making sure the potatoes are cooked but not mushy.

## Baking Casserole

You can reserve some of the cheese to sprinkle on top after you add the milk. The key with this casserole is to cook it to perfection. Too much time and it can easily burn, too little time and your potatoes will get too crunchy. Sample as you go to see how it's doing.

# 14

# Pasta

# Linguini with White Clam Sauce

*You can use canned clams instead of fresh if necessary; just be sure to separate the clams from the juice and save the juice.*

**Yields 4 servings**
Calories: 660
Fat: 18 grams
Protein: 33 grams
Carbohydrates: 92 grams
Cholesterol: 44 milligrams

*3 dozen cherrystone clams*
*¼ cup canola oil*
*¼ cup minced garlic*
*2 tablespoons chopped parsley*
*salt and pepper to taste*
*1 pound whole wheat linguini*

1. Open clams and drain the juice into a small bowl. Reserve juice.

2. Chop clams coarsely with a sharp knife. Set aside.

3. Heat canola oil in a saucepan on medium heat and add clam juice, garlic, and parsley.

4. Simmer for about 30 minutes

5. Add the clams, salt, and pepper. Simmer for 5 more minutes.

6. Cook linguini according to the package directions.

7. Drain linguini and pour sauce over pasta.

8. Mix well and serve.

## Opening Clams

You will need a clam knife to open an uncooked clam. If you don't have one, use a thin, dull kitchen knife. Do not use a sharp knife and have a towel handy to protect your hands while opening the clam. Open clams over a bowl to reserve the clam juice.

The Everything Calorie Counting Cookbook

# Whole Wheat Spaghetti with Jalapeño Tomato Sauce

*Use Romano cheese instead of Parmesan cheese if you prefer.*

1. Cook spaghetti noodles as directed.

2. Combine tomatoes, onions, garlic, bouillon cubes, and jalapeño peppers in a food processor or blender until smooth.

3. Put blended mixture in a large saucepan and heat on medium for about 5 minutes.

*Yields 6 servings;*
*serving size 4 ounces*
Calories: 320
Fat: 3 grams
Protein: 14 grams
Carbohydrates: 65 grams
Cholesterol: 4 milligrams

*1 pound whole wheat spaghetti*
*1 28-ounce can no-sodium diced*
*tomatoes*
*¼ cup minced onions*
*½ teaspoon minced garlic*
*2 low-sodium vegetable bouillon*
*cubes*
*3 jalapeño peppers, diced*
*⅓ cup grated Parmesan cheese*

# Pasta Alfredo

**Yields 6 servings**
Calories: 570
Fat: 24 grams
Protein: 24 grams
Carbohydrates: 61 grams
Cholesterol: 28 milligrams

*1 pound fettuccine noodles*
*½ cup margarine*
*2 cups skim milk*
*⅓ teaspoon nutmeg*
*1⅓ cups freshly grated Parmesan cheese*

If the pasta mixture has become thick and tight, thin it with some of the reserved cooking water.

1. Prepare the fettuccine according to package directions. When pasta is done, drain in a colander and reserve some of the cooking water.

2. Meanwhile, melt margarine in a saucepan over medium heat.

3. Whisk in the milk and nutmeg and bring the mixture to simmer.

4. Add the fettuccine to the cream mixture and top with the cheese.

## Counting Calories

A protein calorie is no different from a fat calorie, they are simply units of energy. However, fat packs more calories per gram than proteins or carbohydrates. The key to weight loss is to burn more calories than you take in.

# Spaghetti with Crab and Corn

This is a truly delicious recipe that you will enjoy serving to your family and friends. To keep it mild, don't add the cayenne pepper.

1. Cook the pasta according to package directions.

2. Heat the vegetable oil in a skillet on medium heat, then add the bacon and cook it until crisp.

3. Remove bacon from skillet and pat with paper towels to remove fat and oils.

4. Sauté onions, celery, bell pepper, and garlic in the leftover oil.

5. Whisk in milk and chicken stock until bubbling., then add the flour and turn the heat down to low.

6. Stir in crab, corn, and cayenne pepper according to taste. Mix well on low heat for about 5 minutes.

7. Add the cheese.

8. Toss entire mixture with drained pasta and serve.

*Yields 6 servings*
Calories: 495
Fat: 11 grams
Protein: 30 grams
Carbohydrates: 77 grams
Cholesterol: 43 milligrams

1 pound whole wheat spaghetti
2 tablespoons vegetable oil
5 slices bacon
2 small onions
3 garlic cloves, crushed
2 stalks celery, finely chopped
½ small red bell pepper, chopped
1 cup low-sodium chicken stock
1 cup nonfat milk
2 tablespoons flour
10 ounces fresh crabmeat
10 ounces frozen corn, thawed
1 teaspoon cayenne pepper
½ cup low-fat shredded cheddar cheese

# Pasta Carbonara

Pancetta is a delicate Italian meat similar to bacon. It can
be cooked in much the same way and is deliciously crispy.

*Yields 6 servings*
Calories: 428
Fat: 11 grams
Protein: 21 grams
Carbohydrates: 57 grams
Cholesterol: 27 milligrams


*1 pound spaghetti*
*½ cup Egg Beaters*
*¼ cup grated Parmesan cheese*
*¼ cup grated Pecorino-Romano*
*cheese*
*Morton's lite salt and cracked*
*pepper to taste*
*½ cup diced pancetta*

1. Cook spaghetti according to package directions.

2. In a mixing bowl, whisk the Egg Beaters, Parmesan, Pecorino, and salt and pepper until it is thick and creamy.

3. Mix the egg mixture and pasta together carefully.

4. Add the pancetta.

### Egg Beaters with Pasta

It is important to make sure the pasta is very hot when added to the egg mixture because it blends better with the pasta to make a creamy coating. If the egg mixture is not hot enough, the sauce will appear chunky.

# Vegetable Pasta

Warm your vegetables in a skillet or in the microwave. If you prefer to cook them for a softer texture, use a skillet and stir them until they are soft or slightly browned.

1. Cook spaghetti according to directions.

2. In a skillet over medium heat, toss the mixed vegetables to warm them.

3. Mix rosemary, onion, garlic, and salt and pepper with the vegetables.

4. Pour vegetables over spaghetti and serve, sprinkling with cheese.

*Yields 6 servings*
Calories: 313
Fat: 2 grams
Protein: 14 grams
Carbohydrates: 64 grams
Cholesterol: 3 milligrams

*1 pound whole wheat spaghetti*
*10 ounces mixed frozen vegetables, thawed*
*2 teaspoons minced onion*
*2 teaspoons minced garlic*
*1 teaspoon freshly grated rosemary*
*salt and pepper to taste*
*¼ cup Parmesan cheese*

# Fresh Tomato with Angel Hair Pasta

### Serves 4–6
Calories: 277
Fat: 18 grams
Protein: 19 grams
Carbohydrates: 25 grams
Cholesterol: 25 milligrams

½ cup pine nuts
4 ripe beefsteak tomatoes
¼ cup extra virgin olive oil
1 tablespoon lemon juice
¼ cup packed fresh basil leaves
½ teaspoon salt
⅛ teaspoon white pepper
1 pound angel hair pasta

This sauce should only be made in the summer when you can find vine-ripened fresh red tomatoes.

1. Bring a large pot of water to a boil for the pasta. Place small skillet over medium heat for 3 minutes. Add pine nuts; cook and stir for 3 to 5 minutes or until nuts begin to brown and are fragrant. Remove from heat and pour nuts into a serving bowl.

2. Chop tomatoes into ½" pieces and add to pine nuts along with olive oil, lemon juice, basil, salt, and pepper. Add pasta to the boiling water; cook and stir until al dente, according to package directions. Drain and add to tomato mixture in bowl. Toss gently and serve immediately.

## Fresh Basil
If you have a garden—or even just a sunny windowsill—by all means grow basil; it's easy to grow and requires very little maintenance. There are lots of kits available on the market or the Internet. Just be sure to use the basil before the plant starts to flower. You can also find fresh basil in the produce aisle of your supermarket.

# Lasagna

*This recipe works well in a 9" x 9" cooking pan.*

1. Cook lasagna noodles according to package directions.

2. Cook zucchini in boiling water for 2 minutes. Drain.

3. Mix cottage cheese, egg white, and mozzarella cheese in a medium bowl. Set aside.

4. Brown beef in a deep skillet and drain.

5. Stir in the spaghetti sauce and fennel. Simmer for 5 minutes.

6. Spay your cooking pan lightly and preheat oven to 350°F.

7. Spread a small amount of the sauce on bottom of cooking pan.

8. Layer the noodles, zucchini, cottage cheese mixture, and sauce in that order.

9. Top with remaining mozzarella.

10. Bake at 350°F for 30 minutes or until lasagna is bubbly and golden brown.

*Yields 6 servings*
Calories: 417
Fat: 6 grams
Protein: 24 grams
Carbohydrates: 70 grams
Cholesterol: 20 milligrams

*1 pound dry lasagna noodles*
*1 medium zucchini, sliced*
*1 cup low-fat cottage cheese*
*1 egg white*
*½ cup skim milk shredded mozzarella cheese*
*¼ pound extra lean ground beef*
*1 jar reduced-sodium chunky vegetable spaghetti sauce*
*½ teaspoon ground fennel*

# Macaroni and Cheese

*Yields 4 servings*
Calories: 368
Fat: 11 grams
Protein: 19 grams
Carbohydrates: 48 grams
Cholesterol: 11 milligrams

*2 cups macaroni noodles*
*½ stalk celery, minced*
*¼ cup onion, minced*
*2 tablespoons canola oil*
*4 tablespoons flour*
*3 tablespoons fat-free milk*
*1 cup of low-fat grated cheddar*
*   cheese*
*½ cup low-fat grated Swiss cheese*
*½ teaspoon grated nutmeg*
*salt and pepper to taste*

There are virtually hundreds of ways to make this macaroni and cheese your own. Using two different cheeses makes the flavor undeniable, but you can stick to one if you prefer.

1. Cook macaroni according to package directions.

2. Sauté minced celery and onion in a skillet with the oil over medium heat.

3. Mix in the milk and flour, stirring until smooth.

4. Mix in the cheese, stirring constantly until thick.

5. Remove immediately from heat.

6. Stir in the nutmeg and season with salt and pepper.

7. Pour mixture over the macaroni. Toss and serve.

## Nutmeg

Nutmeg always adds a slight hint of spice and helps bring out the flavor in cheese sauces. You can use a pinch of pre-ground nutmeg, but fresh nutmeg has much more flavor and aroma. Keep a whole nutmeg in a tiny micrograter made just for that purpose, and grate a bit of fresh nutmeg over everything from cheese sauce to potatoes.

# Broccoli and Noodle Casserole

*If you don't have a casserole dish, any baking dish will do.*
*Just be sure to layer the ingredients evenly.*

1. Preheat oven to 350°F.

2. Cook broccoli in boiling water until tender.

3. Drain broccoli, cool, and cut into 1" pieces.

4. Melt the margarine in a deep skillet on medium heat.

5. Add the flour, milk, and salt and pepper and mix until creamy. Remove from heat and set aside.

6. Boil water and cook the noodles about 15 minutes or until soft, then drain and set aside.

7. In a casserole dish, arrange alternate layers of noodles, broccoli, sliced cooked eggs, cream sauce, and cheese.

8. Sprinkle evenly with bread crumbs.

9. Bake for 30 minutes or until bubbling.

## Versatile Vegetables

You can use nearly any vegetable for this casserole. Asparagus and cauliflower are good alternatives—and there's no rule saying you can only use one vegetable at a time! You can also play around with different cheeses and pastas to find a combination that suits your palate.

*Yields 4 servings*
Calories: 473
Fat: 19 grams
Protein: 23 grams
Carbohydrates: 54 grams
Cholesterol: 216 milligrams

*10 ounces frozen broccoli*
*4 tablespoons margarine*
*4 tablespoons flour*
*2 cups fat-free milk*
*salt and pepper to taste*
*2 cups whole wheat macaroni noodles*
*4 cups of water*
*4 hardboiled eggs*
*¼ cup grated low-fat Swiss cheese*
*1 cup bread crumbs*

# Wild Rice and Onion Pasta

*Caramelized onions and garlic add fabulous flavor to tender pasta
and chewy wild rice. Fresh parsley and basil are the perfect finishing touch.*

**Serves 4**
Calories: 320
Fat: 14 grams
Protein: 16 grams
Carbohydrates: 39 grams
Cholesterol: 45 milligrams

½ cup wild rice
1 cup water
½ pound linguine
1 tablespoon olive oil
2 tablespoons butter
2 onions, chopped
3 cloves garlic, minced
½ cup grated Parmesan cheese
¼ cup chopped parsley
¼ cup chopped fresh basil

1. In a small saucepan, combine wild rice and water. Bring to a boil over high heat, cover, reduce heat, and simmer for 35–40 minutes or until wild rice is tender. Meanwhile, bring a large pot of water to a boil. Add linguine and cook.

2. In heavy saucepan, combine olive oil and butter over medium heat. Add onions and garlic; cook and stir until onions begin to caramelize, about 10–15 minutes.

3. When pasta is done, drain in a colander, reserving about ⅓ cup of the pasta water. Add pasta and reserved water to skillet with onions and reduce heat to low. Add wild rice to skillet; cook and stir for 2 minutes. Sprinkle with cheese, parsley, and basil. Stir and serve immediately.

# 15

# Meat Accompaniments and Sauces

# Tartar Sauce

This is good for an appetizer sauce and excellent with
scallops, shrimp, fish, cold cuts, and cold chicken.

1. Beat canola oil and white vinegar. Add scallion tops, mayonnaise, and egg yolk
   mixture. Beat until smooth.

## Tartar Sauce History
Tartar sauce was invented by the French, who served it with raw steak. Over time, this raw
steak became known as Steak Tartare because of the Tartar sauce.

### Yields 26 servings
Calories: 84
Fat: 9 grams
Protein: 0 grams
Carbohydrates: 0 grams
Cholesterol: 17 milligrams

1 cup canola oil
5 tablespoons white vinegar
2 hardboiled egg yolks
1 tablespoon scallion tops, chopped
2 tablespoons low-fat mayonnaise

# Beef Horseradish

You can add a few drops of hot pepper sauce to this recipe if you want it more tangy.

1. Combine all ingredients in medium bowl and blend well. Chill until ready to
   serve.

### Yields 40 servings
Calories: 13
Fat: 0 grams
Protein:<1 gram
Carbohydrates: 2 grams
Cholesterol: 1 milligram

2 cups fat-free sour cream
¼ cup horseradish, drained
1 teaspoon minced chives
1 teaspoon white wine vinegar
salt and pepper to taste

# Basil Pesto Sauce

You can warm the pine nuts for a few minutes under the broiler before
you add them to the recipe, which gives you a different, toasty flavor.

1. Pour all ingredients except the oil into a food processor and blend until it
   forms a paste. Gradually blend in oil and adjust seasonings to taste.

### Presto! It's Pesto!

Pesto sauce has been around since the Romans and is actually any combination of herbs
crushed and mixed with oil. In the old days, cooks used a mortar and pestle to make this
uncooked basil sauce, but a food processor works just as well.

*Yields 15 servings;*
*serving size 1 tablespoon*
Calories: 71
Fat: 8 grams
Protein: <1 gram
Carbohydrates: <1 gram
Cholesterol: 1 milligram

*1½ teaspoons minced garlic*
*2 cups coarsely chopped basil leaves*
*¼ teaspoon pine nuts*
*3 tablespoons Parmesan cheese*
*½ cup olive oil*

# Baked Fish Sauce

This sauce is best when poured over fish and baked in the oven for 20 minutes.

1. Melt butter in a deep skillet over medium heat.

2. Add in the onion and flour, mixing as you go.

3. Add the cheese and milk. Cook until cheese is melted and sauce is thick.

*Yields 27 servings*
Calories: 20
Fat: 2 grams
Protein: 1 gram
Carbohydrates: 1 gram
Cholesterol: 4 milligrams

*1 tablespoon butter*
*1 onion, chopped*
*1 tablespoon flour*
*3 slices American cheese*
*1½ cups skim milk*

# Mushroom Sauce

The soup stock should be cold when added to this recipe.

**Yields 27 servings**
Calories: 10
Fat: 1 gram
Protein: <1 gram
Carbohydrates: <1 gram
Cholesterol: 2 milligrams

2 tablespoons light butter
2 tablespoons flour
1 cup low-sodium meat or
vegetable stock, chilled
4 tablespoons half-n-half
salt and pepper to taste
½ cup mushrooms, chopped and
sautéed

1. Heat butter and flour in a deep skillet over medium heat until smooth; allow to brown.

2. Add stock, stirring constantly. When sauce is smooth, bring to a boil. Cook for 3 minutes.

3. Add half-n-half, salt, and pepper, mixing as you add. Add mushrooms and blend until heated. Remove from flame and serve.


# Faux Sour Cream

This sauce has all the flavor and creaminess of a thick sour cream without the guilt in calories!

**Yields 6 servings**
Calories: 12
Fat: < 1 gram
Protein: 1 gram
Carbohydrates: 1 gram
Cholesterol: 1 milligram

⅛ cup plain nonfat yogurt
¼ cup cottage cheese
½ teaspoon vinegar

1. Put all the ingredients in a blender or food processor; process until smooth.

### Vinegar Options
The type of vinegar used in the Faux Sour Cream recipe will affect the "tang" of the sour cream taste. Apple cider vinegar, for example, has a stronger taste; white wine or champagne vinegar tends to be milder.

# Red Wine Butter Sauce

A dry red wine is the best for this recipe because it tastes best with the beef stock.

1. Sauté butter and flour until smooth in a deep skillet over medium heat.

2. Blend in wine. Blend in beef stock. Thicken sauce, then remove from heat and serve.

*Yields 18 servings*
Calories: 13
Fat: 1 gram
Protein: 0 grams
Carbohydrates: 1 gram
Cholesterol: 2 milligrams

*1 tablespoon flour*
*1 tablespoon butter*
*½ cup red wine*
*½ cup low-sodium beef stock*

# Sour Cream Dill Sauce

It is important to mix ingredients well before adding in
new ones to make sure your sauce doesn't get lumpy.

1. Heat butter in a deep skillet over medium heat. Blend in flour until smooth. After browning slightly, blend in soup stock.

2. After sauce is smooth, bring to boiling point. Lower heat and cook for 3 minutes.

3. Add cream and blend well; add dill and blend until heated through. Remove from heat, add salt and pepper to your tasting, and serve.

*Yields 36 servings*
Calories: 14
Fat: 1 gram
Protein: 1 gram
Carbohydrates: 1 gram
Cholesterol: 3 milligrams

*1 tablespoon butter*
*1 tablespoon all-purpose flour, sifted*
*1 cup low-sodium chicken stock*
*1 cup low-fat sour cream*
*salt and pepper to taste*
*1½ tablespoons fresh dill, chopped*

### Dill and Salmon
Dill and salmon make a heavenly combination. Serve this sauce with thin slices of smoked salmon by themselves or bundle them into a crepe for a filling meal. This recipe is tasty and healthier than the heavy cream cheese and salmon you can order at the deli.

# Parmesan Dressing

Use freshly squeezed lemon juice in this recipe with
freshly grated cheese to make the flavors truly pop.

**Yields 14 servings**
Calories: 49
Fat: 4 grams
Protein: 2 grams
Carbohydrates: 1 gram
Cholesterol: 3 milligrams

3 tablespoons extra virgin olive oil
2 teaspoons minced garlic
3 tablespoons white wine
3 tablespoons fresh lemon juice
2 tablespoons Splenda
½ cup freshly grated Parmesan
    cheese

1. Warm the olive oil in a deep skillet.

2. Add in the garlic, white wine, lemon juice, and Splenda.

3. Cook on medium heat for about 3 minutes.

4. Blend in grated Parmesan cheese and cook for 2 minutes before serving over salad, chicken, or rice.

# Artichoke Pesto

You can use freshly picked basil and thyme for a zestier flavor, but bottled seasoning is okay.

**Yields 48 servings**
Calories: 37
Fat: 4 grams
Protein: 0 grams
Carbohydrates: 1 gram
Cholesterol: 0 milligrams

¾ cup canola oil
3 teaspoons minced garlic
⅓ cup lemon juice
1 teaspoon crushed thyme
1 bay leaf
salt and pepper to taste
1 14-ounce can artichoke hearts
½ cup packed fresh basil leaves,
    chopped

1. Preheat oven to 350°F.

2. Combine ½ cup oil, lemon juice, garlic, thyme, bay leaf, salt, and pepper in a medium bowl. Add artichoke hearts and mix. Transfer ingredients to a deep skillet and cook over stove until boiling, stirring occasionally.

3. Transfer ingredients to an ovenproof dish or bake pan, cover with foil and put into oven for 30 minutes. Allow mixture to cool and remove bay leaf.

4. Put all ingredients into blender with ¼ cup oil and basil leaves. Blend until smooth.

### Pesto Uses

This pesto tastes excellent spread over toasted ciabatta bread or mixed in with any type of pasta. Try baking homemade pizza with pesto sauce instead of tomato sauce for a tangier flavor. Commercial pesto sauce is easy to find in grocery stores, but it's almost as easy to make your own; making your own also gives you control over the ingredients and the calorie count.

# 16

# Salads

# Flank Steak Salad

**Yields 4 servings**
Calories: 253
Fat: 15 grams
Protein: 25 grams
Carbohydrates: 4 grams
Cholesterol: 40 milligrams

*1 pound flank steak, thinly sliced*
*salt and pepper to taste*
*1 tablespoon canola oil*
*1 teaspoon garlic, minced*
*1 teaspoon oregano*
*2 tablespoons red wine vinegar*
*1 tablespoon margarine*
*1 12-ounce bag Italian salad blend*

*To save time, have your flank steak sliced at the meat counter in the grocery store.*

1. Season the flank steak pieces with salt and pepper.

2. Heat the canola oil in a skillet. Sauté flank steak pieces until cooked through.

3. Stir in the garlic, oregano, and vinegar.

4. Add the margarine to the skillet and let it melt.

5. Add the salad greens to the skillet. Stir for about 30 seconds.

6. Transfer all ingredients to a plate and serve.

The Everything Calorie Counting Cookbook

# Chunky Chicken Salad

Use leftover chicken or buy pre-cut chicken to save time.

1. Combine all ingredients in a salad bowl. Cover and refrigerate.

### Fill Up on Salad

Salad can be very filling, especially when it is served with a protein like chicken. Hearty salads can replace meaty meals. It's a good way to ensure you get enough protein and vegetables. Tucking your salad in whole wheat pita bread takes care of a serving of grains as well.

*Yields 4 servings*
Calories: 325
Fat: 16 grams
Protein: 33 grams
Carbohydrates: 12 grams
Cholesterol: 105 milligrams

*1 pound cooked white chicken meat, cut into 1" slices*
*1 cup finely diced celery*
*½ cup finely diced sweet onion*
*3 tablespoons sweet relish*
*½ cup fat-free Miracle Whip salad dressing*
*salt and pepper to taste*

# Salmon Salad

*You can use canned salmon for this recipe. Don't worry
if the fresh fish or the canned fish has bones.*

1. Combine all ingredients. Mix well and serve cold.

## Serving Salmon Salad

If you would prefer, you can always grill a salmon steak instead of mixing salmon with the salad. After grilling, serve the salmon atop the salad fixings and garnish with sauce or diced vegetables like red peppers. For more zing, marinate the salmon in the sauce you will use to dress the salad.

*Yields 2 servings*
Calories: 580
Fat: 33 grams
Protein: 59 grams
Carbohydrates: 10 grams
Cholesterol: 160 milligrams

2 cups cooked salmon
1 cup celery, finely diced
½ cup sweet white or red onion,
 finely diced
2 tablespoons fresh dill, minced
1 green pepper, finely diced
1 teaspoon fennel seed
2 tablespoons white wine vinegar
2 tablespoons canola oil
salt and pepper to taste

# Tomato and Onion Salad

To remove skin from tomatoes, place them in boiling water for 30 seconds. Take a paring knife and slice an "X" into the skin at the bottom of the tomato. The skins will come off easily.

1. Cut up peeled tomatoes into 1" cubes, removing seeds.

2. Finely slice the onion, halving the rings.

3. Combine the tomato wedges and the onion slices.

4. Add basil, oil, vinegar, salt, pepper, and Splenda.

5. Cover and refrigerate for 20 minutes before serving.

## Marinating Basics

Allowing ingredients to sit and marinate lets the juices in and enhances the flavor. It's a good idea to do this whenever you're using oils, pepper, and salt on non-leafy vegetables. Tomatoes and onions are perfect candidates for marinating, but spinach, for instance, will turn soggy.

**_Yields 4 servings_**
Calories: 200
Fat: 19 grams
Protein: 1 gram
Carbohydrates: 6 grams
Cholesterol: 0 milligrams

2 large ripe tomatoes, peeled
1 large Vidalia onion
1 teaspoon fresh basil
⅓ cup canola oil
4 tablespoons cider vinegar
1 tablespoon Splenda
salt and pepper to taste

# Cucumber and Red Onion Salad

You can use 2 large seedless cucumbers instead of regular ones to save time.

_Yields 4 servings_
Calories: 288
Fat: 28 grams
Protein: 1 gram
Carbohydrates: 10 grams
Cholesterol: 0 milligrams

2 large cucumbers
2 cups water
1 large red onion, sliced into thin
    rings
¼ cup cider vinegar
½ cup canola oil
salt and pepper to taste
1 teaspoon Splenda

1. Peel cucumbers, halve them, and scoop out the seeds.

2. Slice cucumber and and place in a bowl with salted water for 20 minutes.

3. Drain cucumber slices.

4. Combine cucumber slices and onion slices.

5. Add the rest of the ingredients; refrigerate until ready to serve.

# Sinfully Thin Salad

Boston lettuce is best with this recipe because it is
both light and buttery, hence its nickname, "butter" lettuce.

1. Wash, dry, and separate leaves of Boston lettuce.

2. Combine lettuce with the rest of the ingredients.

3. Serve immediately.

## Serving Lettuce

It's not a good idea to marinate anything with lettuce because the leaves will take on too much water and oil and get soggy. Dress the lettuce immediately before serving or leave the salad naked and let people add as much or as little dressing as they like.

*Yields 4 servings*
Calories: 213
Fat: 22 grams
Protein: 2 grams
Carbohydrates: 4 grams
Cholesterol: 0 milligrams

*1 head Boston lettuce*
*2 tablespoons artificial bacon pieces*
*1 teaspoon Splenda*
*4 tablespoons red wine vinegar*
*6 tablespoons canola oil*
*salt and pepper to taste*

# Dilled Tomato and Onion Salad

**_Yields 4 servings_**
Calories: 143
Fat: 11 grams
Protein: 2 grams
Carbohydrates: 11 grams
Cholesterol: 0 milligrams

*4 large tomatoes, thinly sliced*
*1 large Vidalia or sweet onion,*
   *thinly sliced*
*1 tablespoon fresh dill, snipped into*
   *little pieces*
*3 tablespoons canola oil*
*1 tablespoon distilled vinegar*
*1 teaspoon Splenda*
*salt and pepper to taste*

*Peel the tomatoes or leave the peel on depending on your personal preference.*

1. Alternate tomato and onion slices on a platter.

2. Mix the rest of the ingredients and pour over the tomato and onion slices.

3. Cover and refrigerate until cool.

## Sweet Vidalia

Vidalia onions are so sweet that many people eat them whole, like an apple. Some recommend putting some sugar on before you take a bite. They are a good source of vitamin C, and they are low in fat, sodium, cholesterol, and calories. Store them apart from other fruits and vegetables in a cool, dark area.

# Southwestern Corn Salad

*Drain your corn well to avoid excess liquid.*

1. Combine corn, cucumbers, onions, and tomatoes in a salad bowl.

2. Separately combine the rest of the ingredients.

3. Add the dressing to the salad and toss.

4. Cover and refrigerate until cooled.

## Summer Salads

Summer salads, especially those with fresh corn and onions, are best served cold. They don't require much in the way of preparation, and you can be assured of a cool, refreshing salad. During the summer months, take advantage of the wide variety of fresh vegetables at your local market.

*Yields 4 servings*
Calories: 383
Fat: 29 grams
Protein: 5 grams
Carbohydrates: 32 grams
Cholesterol: 1 milligrams

2 cups frozen or canned corn
¾ cup cucumber, seeded and diced
½ cup red onion, minced
1 14-ounce can diced tomatoes
6 scallions, chopped
4 tablespoons nonfat sour cream
¼ cup cider vinegar
½ cup canola oil
salt and pepper to taste

# Pear and Watercress Salad

Chunky bleu cheese is the only type to serve with this salad.

**_Yields 4 servings_**
Calories: 198
Fat: 15 grams
Protein: 4 grams
Carbohydrates: 14 grams
Cholesterol: 11 milligrams

_2 pears_
_3 tablespoons canola oil_
_1½ tablespoons apple cider vinegar_
_salt and pepper to taste_
_1 teaspoon whole-grain mustard_
_½ cup watercress, washed, dried, stems trimmed_
_1 cup arugula, washed, dried, stems trimmed_
_2 ounces bleu cheese, crumbled_

1. Core the pears. Cut into ¾" slices.

2. In 1 teaspoon of canola oil, sauté the pears until brown.

3. Mix the remaining oil with the vinegar, salt, and pepper.

4. Add mustard, whisking until dressing is slightly thick.

5. Mix watercress and arugula in a plastic bag.

6. Put into salad bowl; add bleu cheese.

7. Add pears to salad bowl. Serve immediately.

# Simple Tomato and Mozzarella Salad

You can purchase a vinaigrette dressing or make your own from one of the choices in Chapter 17.

1. Arrange tomato slices and mozzarella slices on a plate, alternating between the two.

2. Pour vinaigrette dressing over slices.

3. Cover, refrigerate, and serve when chilled.

## Dressing Tomatoes

You can use nearly any type of dressing on tomatoes, but most people prefer an oil and vinegar or Italian dressing. For a very simple dressing that goes nicely with tomatoes and mozzarella, mix equal parts extra virgin olive oil and balsamic vinegar and sprinkle with freshly ground black pepper. Garnish with fresh basil leaves.

*Yields 4 servings*
Calories 655
Fat: 53 grams
Protein: 31 grams
Carbohydrates: 14 grams
Cholesterol: 61 milligrams

*4 large beefsteak tomatoes, washed and cut into ½" slices*
*1 pound of skim mozzarella cheese, cut into ½" slices*
*1 cup vinaigrette*

# Crispy Cobb Salad

**Yields 4 servings**
Calories: 303
Fat: 17 grams
Protein: 29 grams
Carbohydrates: 8 grams
Cholesterol: 166 milligrams

4 ounces arugula
2 cups shredded white meat
    chicken, boiled
1 large tomato
2 hardboiled eggs, finely chopped
1 ripe avocado, pitted and sliced
    into small pieces
3 slices cooked bacon
½ cup bottled low-calorie bleu
    cheese dressing

*You can buy chicken already shredded. Vary the dressing with any creamy choice.*

1. Layer shallow salad bowl as follows: arugula, chicken, tomato, eggs, avocado and bacon.

2. Cover with blue cheese dressing and serve immediately.

## Chopping vs. Layering

Many people prefer their salad chopped as opposed to layered. Layering is a fun and different way to serve a salad, with a surprise as you dig in. It also provides a nicer, more ordered presentation, and it's easy to prepare since you don't have to fuss over mixing the salad perfectly.

# Crunchy Macaroni Salad

Add a diced tomato for color if you like. It provides
a touch of fiber with a negligible amount of calories.

1. Mix all ingredients together.

2. Cover, refrigerate until cold, and serve.

### Munching Macaroni

Cook the macaroni *al dente* so it's still chewy. *Al dente* is an Italian term meaning "to the tooth"—firm. A firmer pasta adds a great texture to salad. Pasta can also be cooked *al dente* for casseroles where the noodles will cook further in the oven.

**Yields 4 servings**
Calories: 275
Fat: 9 grams
Protein: 11 grams
Carbohydrates: 36 grams
Cholesterol: 5 milligrams

2 cups elbow macaroni, cooked
   according to package directions
⅓ cup diced celery
⅓ cup finely chopped Vidalia onion
⅔ cup Miracle Whip salad dressing
⅔ cup dry mustard
1 teaspoon Splenda
3 tablespoons fat-free sour cream
salt and pepper to taste

# Crabmeat and Shrimp Salad

Make sure your seafood is thoroughly cooked before mixing
this salad. Serve the salad by itself or on whole wheat buns.

1. Combine all ingredients. Cover salad and refrigerate until chilled. Serve salad on iceberg lettuce leaves.

*Yields 4 servings*

Calories: 170

Fat: 2 grams

Protein: 32 grams

Carbohydrates: 7 grams

Cholesterol: 173 milligrams

¾ pound lump crabmeat, cooked

½ pound shrimp, cooked and diced

4 teaspoons dried chives

1 stalk celery, diced

¼ cup fat-free sour cream

1 teaspoon lemon juice

1 teaspoon Dijon mustard

salt and pepper to taste

1 teaspoon Splenda

1 head iceberg lettuce

The Everything Calorie Counting Cookbook

# Asian Beef Salad

*You can use regular cucumbers in this recipe if you de-seed them first.*

1. Preheat broiler.

2. Broil flank steak strip for 5 minutes on each side.

3. Mix lime juice, fish sauce, Splenda, and chilies in a bowl.

4. Add the scallions, coriander, cucumber, and steak to the dressing.

5. Arrange on a platter and garnish with mint leaves; serve.

## Mint Leaves

Mint makes a good herb garden staple. It can be used to add zip to bland recipes and garnish everything from desserts to salads. Mint leaves have been used as a garnish since the early 1920s because they add an irresistible zest to a variety of flavors. They are also used to garnish cocktails.

*Yields 4 servings*
Calories: 150
Fat: 6 grams
Protein: 19 grams
Carbohydrates: 4 grams
Cholesterol: 30 milligrams

¾ pound flank steak, thinly sliced
    and rolled in black pepper
3 tablespoons lime juice
1 tablespoon Asian fish sauce
½ teaspoon Splenda
1 green Thai chili, seeded and
    minced
2 scallions, diced
2 teaspoons coriander, crushed
½ seedless cucumber, diced
1 teaspoon mint leaves, finely
    chopped

# Hollywood Lobster Salad

**Yields 4 servings**
Calories: 225
Fat: 15 grams
Protein: 18 grams
Carbohydrates: 6 grams
Cholesterol: 63 milligrams

¾ pound lobster meat, cooked and
    torn into chunks
4 tablespoons extra virgin olive oil
1 teaspoon lemon juice
3 tablespoons chopped chives
⅓ cup fat-free Miracle Whip salad
    dressing
salt and pepper to taste
1 head Boston lettuce

You can use any kind of salad greens for this bed of lobster salad,
but the Boston lettuce gives the dish a soft taste and texture.

1.  Gently fold all ingredients except the lettuce together.

2.  Cover and refrigerate until chilled.

3.  Arrange salad on a bed of salad greens and serve immediately.

# Greek Salad

This salad tastes best cold and crispy, so make sure all ingredients are chilled before making it.

1. Lightly toss romaine lettuce with 2 tablespoons dressing.

2. Divide lettuce onto 4 plates.

3. Scatter the rest of the ingredients on top of the lettuce and serve.

## Greek Salad

Greek Salad is traditionally any salad with Grecian-inspired ingredients. Depending on what part of the country you draw your inspiration from, you might find peppercorns, radishes, and even beets in a Greek salad. The key ingredient that all Greek salads have, however, is olive oil and vinegar.

*Yields 4 servings*
Calories: 410
Fat: 34 grams
Protein: 11 grams
Carbohydrates: 17 grams
Cholesterol: 50 milligrams

1 head romaine lettuce, cut into
    small pieces
2 tablespoons Greek salad dressing
1 cup kalamata olives, pitted
½ pound crumbled Feta cheese
1 seedless cucumber, cut into bite-
    sized chunks
1 cup cherry tomatoes
1 medium red onion, diced
1 green pepper, diced
salt and pepper to taste

# Asian Salad

**Yields 4 servings**
Calories: 188
Fat: 8 grams
Protein: 19 grams
Carbohydrates: 10 grams
Cholesterol: 49 milligrams

½ pound chicken meat, cooked and
  shredded
1 cup water chestnuts, drained and
  sliced
4 scallions, diced
3 tablespoons bottled oil and
  vinegar dressing
2 teaspoons low-sodium soy sauce
½ teaspoon ground ginger
3 ounces arugula, stems trimmed

You can use either bottled oil and vinegar dressing, homemade dressing, or a vinaigrette dressing.

1. Place chicken, water chestnuts, and scallions in a bowl.

2. Mix dressing, soy sauce, and ginger.

3. Pour dressing mixture over chicken mixture; toss well.

4. Arrange mixture over greens and serve.

# 17

# Salad Dressings

# Buttermilk Dressing

**_Yields 8 servings_**
Calories: 91
Fat: <1 gram
Protein: 8 grams
Carbohydrates: 12 grams
Cholesterol: 5 milligrams

1 16-ounce carton fat-free cottage
    cheese
2 cups low-fat buttermilk
1 tablespoon chives
1 8-ounce package ranch-style
    salad dressing mix
¼ teaspoon Splenda

Make sure to shake ingredients thoroughly before serving. If you use a blender, blend on low.

1. Combine ingredients in a blender or a container with a cover.

2. Shake or blend until well mixed.

3. Keep refrigerated until ready to pour over salad greens.

### DIY Dressings

Making a dressing is the simplest of all recipes because you do not need sophisticated utensils to create it. If you do not have a mixer or blender, simply put everything in a resealable plastic bag or reusable plastic container and shake until everything is well mixed.

# Cucumber Dressing

*Using Morton's lite salt instead of regular salt decreases sodium content by almost half but keeps the flavor of regular salt*

1. Mix cucumber, vinegar, salt, and pepper in a medium bowl.

2. Cover and let stand for an hour.

3. After an hour, uncover cucumber mixture and fold in mayonnaise and remaining ingredients.

4. Pour over crisp Boston lettuce or mixed salad greens.

<u>*Yields 4 servings*</u>
Calories: 43
Fat: 1 gram
Protein: <1 gram
Carbohydrates: 9 grams
Cholesterol: 4 milligrams

*2 tablespoons finely chopped cucumbers*
*2 tablespoons white vinegar*
*½ teaspoon Morton's lite salt*
*½ teaspoon white pepper*
*½ cup fat-free mayonnaise*
*¼ cup chili sauce*
*1 tablespoon finely chopped celery*
*1 tablespoon finely chopped green pepper*
*1 teaspoon finely chopped onion*

# Lemon and Oil Dressing

**_Yields 4 servings_**
Calories: 183
Fat: 20 grams
Protein: 0 grams
Carbohydrates: 1 gram
Cholesterol: 0 milligrams

6 tablespoons olive oil
2 tablespoons lemon juice
¼ teaspoon Morton's lite salt
1 teaspoon Splenda blended sugar
1 teaspoon Hungarian paprika

The sugar substitute Stevia can be used instead of Splenda, and this will reduce the calories even further, as blended Splenda sugar contains regular sugar.

1. Combine all ingredients in a bottle with a cap and shake well.

## History of Salad Dressing

Salad dressing is the modern adaptation of simple sauce, and sauces date back to ancient times. The Chinese have been using soy sauce in their cooking for more than 5,000 years, and the Babylonians used oil and vinegar more than 2,000 years ago. Romans would dress their salads with salt, while Egyptians preferred oil, vinegar, and Oriental spices.

# Lemon and Honey Dressing

This dressing is a perfect sauce for baked chicken or fish. You can use it as a marinade or pour over the meat once cooked.

1. Mix lemon juice and honey in a small bowl.

2. Add the nutmeg and salt and continue to whisk briskly.

3. Serve over salad.

*Yields 2 servings*
Calories: 180
Fat: 0 grams
Protein: <1 gram
Carbohydrates: 50 grams
Cholesterol: 0 milligrams

¼ cup lemon juice
⅓ cup honey
¼ teaspoon nutmeg
¼ teaspoon salt

# Lemon-Mustard Dressing

*This dressing is equally good for fresh salad greens or a bed of lettuce with slices of apples and mandarin oranges.*

**_Yields 2 servings_**
Calories: 18
Fat: <1 gram
Protein: <1 gram
Carbohydrates: 4 grams
Cholesterol: 0 milligrams

¼ cup lemon juice
1 teaspoon dry mustard
1 teaspoon Morton's lite salt
¼ teaspoon white pepper
1 teaspoon Splenda

1. Combine all ingredients in a jar with a lid and shake well.

2. Refrigerate for 1 hour before serving.

## Cold Dressings

Some dressings are fine served at room temperature, but this one is best served very cold. It makes the mustard snap and stand out in the dressing.

# No-Oil Salad Dressing

You can buy minced onion and garlic in jars in the vegetable
section of your food store to save having to mince or chop your own.

1. Combine Splenda, mustard, lite salt, paprika, and pepper.

2. Slowly add vinegar to the mixture.

3. Add tomato soup, Worcestershire sauce, onion, and garlic.

4. Store dressing in refrigerator.

5. Shake well each time you use the dressing.

*Yields 8 servings*
Calories: 55
Fat: <1 gram
Protein: <1 gram
Carbohydrates: 13 grams
Cholesterol: 0 milligrams

⅓ cup Splenda
1 teaspoon dry mustard
1 teaspoon Morton's lite salt
½ teaspoon sweet paprika
½ teaspoon pepper
⅓ cup white vinegar
1 10-ounce can low-sodium tomato
   soup
1 tablespoon Worcestershire sauce
1 tablespoon onion, finely minced
1 clove garlic, finely minced

# Faux Sour Cream Dressing

**Yields 6 servings**
Calories: 35
Fat: 2 grams
Protein: 2 grams
Carbohydrates: 3 grams
Cholesterol: 7 milligrams

*1 teaspoon flour*
*1¼ teaspoon dry mustard*
*¼ cup Splenda*
*Morton's lite salt to taste*
*¼ cup water*
*¾ cup vinegar*
*¼ cup Egg Beaters*
*2 tablespoons lite butter*

The Egg Beaters keep the calories down, but you can use two whole eggs, beaten, if you prefer. Just remember to add the calories in to your overall day count.

1. Mix flour, mustard, Splenda, and salt in a large saucepan together. Add water, vinegar, and Egg Beaters. Cook over medium heat until the mixture thickens.

2. Add butter. Cook until mixture thickens.

3. Remove from stove. Let cool for several minutes.

4. Beat well until smooth and creamy.

5. Store in glass jar with cover until ready for use.

### Mayonnaise Substitute
You can make this a mayonnaise dressing if you prefer. Just add ¼ cup of vegetable oil. Your homemade mayonnaise dressing will be lower in sugar and sodium than commercial products. Early mayonnaise was nothing more than egg yolks, oil, and seasoning.

# Fresh Tomato Dressing

This is perfect over shrimp, drizzled onto avocados, or even used
as a sauce for hot or cold chicken or fish. It tastes summery!

1. Puree all ingredients in the blender. Taste for salt and pepper. This dressing
   improves with age—try making it a day or two in advance.

## Balsamic Vinegar

There are various types of Italian vinegar, but perhaps the most famous is balsamic vinegar.
Balsamic vinegar is made from reduced wine and aged in special wood barrels for years. Each
year's barrels are made of a different type of wood—the vinegar absorbs the flavor of the
wood. Authentic balsamic vinegar ages for a minimum of 10 and up to 30 years.

### Yields 16 servings
Calories: 78
Fat: 7 grams
Protein: 0 grams
Carbohydrates: 2 milligrams

1 pint basket cherry tomatoes
4 cloves roasted garlic
2 shallots
2 jalapeño peppers, cored and
    seeded
¼ cup stemmed, loosely packed
    fresh basil
¼ cup red wine or balsamic vinegar
½ cup extra virgin olive oil
½ teaspoon celery salt
2 teaspoons Worcestershire sauce
freshly ground black pepper to taste
½ teaspoon cayenne pepper or to
    taste

# Caesar Dressing

True Caesar salad dressing has a touch of anchovy, lemon, and mustard.

**Yields 8 servings**
Calories: 83
Fat: 9 grams
Protein: 2 grams
Carbohydrates: 0 milligrams

¼ cup red wine vinegar
1 raw pasteurized egg
1 clove garlic, mashed
1 tablespoon lemon juice
½ teaspoon dry English mustard
½ inch anchovy paste
salt and pepper to taste
¼ cup freshly grated Parmesan
   cheese
¼ cup olive oil
parsley for garnish

1.  Puree the vinegar, egg, garlic, and lemon juice in a blender. Add the mustard, anchovy paste, salt, pepper, and cheese.

2.  With the motor running, slowly add the olive oil in a thin stream. Garnish with fresh parsley to taste.

### Which Olive Oil Is Best?

Extra virgin olive oil comes from the first pressing of the olives, has the most intense flavor, and is the most expensive. Use this for salads and for dressings and dips. Virgin olive oil is from the second pressing. Less expensive than extra virgin, it can be used for the same purposes. If the label says simply "olive oil" it indicates that it is from the last pressing; this is the oil used for cooking since it does not burn as easily at high temperatures.

# Yogurt and Herb (Ranch)

*This tastes delicious with vegetables.*

1. Whisk all ingredients together and serve.

*Yields 8 servings*
Calories: 17
Fat: 0 grams
Protein: 1 gram
Carbohydrates: 2 grams
Cholesterol: 2 milligrams

*1 cup low-fat yogurt*
*2 tablespoons lemon juice*
*2 tablespoons chopped chives*
*½ teaspoon celery salt*
*½ teaspoon garlic powder*
*2 drops Tabasco sauce or to taste*

# Onion Dressing

**Yields 4 servings**
Calories: 260
Fat: 28 grams
Protein: <1 gram
Carbohydrates: 3 grams
Cholesterol: 0 milligrams

½ cup minced red onion
⅓ cup chopped parsley
2 tablespoons cider vinegar
Morton's lite salt and pepper to
    taste
½ cup canola oil

*Be sure to use a red onion for this dressing because it has more punch than a white onion. It also adds some nice color to the overall presentation.*

1. Combine all ingredients in a blender and blend until mixture is uniform.

2. Store covered in a glass container in refrigerator until ready to use.

### Commercial Dressings

It was unheard of to actually buy salad dressing in a grocery store until the turn of the twentieth century. Restaurants were actually the first to create and package their own salad dressings and the industry caught on from there.

# Creamy Cheese and Buttermilk Dressing

*Sago cheese or gorgonzola cheese can be substituted for the bleu in the recipe.*

1. Place the buttermilk, mustard, garlic powder, and Worcestershire sauce in a blender and blend until smooth.

2. Add sour cream and pulse blend until smooth.

3. Crumble cheese into small bits and place in blender; blend at low speed for 3 minutes.

**_Yields 6 servings_**
Calories: 107
Fat: 6 grams
Protein: 7 grams
Carbohydrates: 6 grams
Cholesterol: 18 milligrams

1 cup buttermilk
½ teaspoon dry mustard
½ teaspoon garlic powder
1 teaspoon Worcestershire sauce
½ cup fat-free sour cream
4 ounces imported Danish bleu
    cheese

# Fresh Mint Vinegar Dressing

*If you like the tart flavor, add a little lime juice to this recipe.*

*Yields 6 servings*
Calories: 93
Fat: 9 grams
Protein: <1 gram
Carbohydrates: 3 grams
Cholesterol: 0 milligrams

*¼ cup freshly squeezed orange juice*
*⅓ cup freshly squeezed lemon juice*
*1 teaspoon salt*
*1 teaspoon pepper*
*1 garlic clove, crushed*
*¼ cup canola oil*
*½ cup flat-leaf parsley*
*½ cup fresh mint leaves*

1. Whisk together lemon juice, orange juice, salt, and pepper.

2. Drizzle canola oil into juice mixture and whisk until well blended.

3. Wash and dry parsley and mint and put into a salad bowl.

4. Add the garlic and the blended dressing.

5. Toss to coat leaves evenly.

6. Place in glass jar with cover and store until needed.

## Salad Days

The term "salad days" was first coined by playwright William Shakespeare. In *Antony and Cleopatra*, Cleopatra regrets her affair with Julius Caesar. Pleading with her new love, Antony, she explains the tryst with Caesar took place in "My salad days, / When I was green in judgment, cold in blood." Today we still use the term to refer to a time of youthful inexperience.

# Lime French Dressing

If you're not a fan of the lime, substitute a lemon instead.

1. Measure all ingredients into a glass bottle with cover.

2. Shake well.

3. Refrigerate until ready to use.

**Yields 4 servings**
Calories: 188
Fat: 21 grams
Protein: 0 grams
Carbohydrates: 1 gram
Cholesterol: 0 milligrams

6 tablespoons canola oil
2 tablespoons lime juice
¼ teaspoon Morton's lite salt
1 teaspoon Splenda
¼ teaspoon paprika

# 18

# Sandwiches,
# Wraps, and Melts

# Mama's Egg Salad Sandwich

*These ingredients must be well mixed to make the egg salad easy to spread.*

**Yields 4 servings**
Calories: 283
Fat: 11 grams
Protein: 15 grams
Carbohydrates: 32 grams
Cholesterol: 321 milligrams

*6 hardboiled eggs*
*½ cup fat-free Miracle Whip salad*
*dressing*
*¼ cup finely chopped celery*
*2 tablespoons finely chopped flat-*
*leaf parsley*
*salt and pepper to taste*

1. Separate the hardboiled egg whites from the yolks. Finely chop egg whites.

2. Press egg yolks through a sieve and add to chopped egg whites in small bowl.

3. Add salad dressing, celery, and parsley and blend well. Season with salt and pepper to taste.

4. Chill mixture for one hour. Spread on your favorite bread.

# Bacon, Lettuce, and Tomato Sandwich

This sandwich is commonly known as the "BLT" and is usually made with white bread, but some brands of whole wheat bread have fewer calories. Wheat bread usually contains more fiber. Select whole grain bread for the most nutrition.

1. Broil the bacon. Spread a thin layer of Miracle Whip on pieces of toasted bread. Arrange bacon and tomato slices on toast with crisp lettuce.

## The BLT

It is not known who coined the term BLT, but the term appears in cookbooks dating back to the 1930s, when it was typically made with cheese.

---

*Yields 4 servings*
Calories: 245
Fat: 8 grams
Protein: 12 grams
Carbohydrates: 35 grams
Cholesterol: 14 milligrams

6 slices extra lean bacon
4 teaspoons fat-free Miracle Whip
    salad dressing
8 slices whole wheat bread, toasted
2 large tomatoes, thinly sliced
1 head of lettuce

# Crabmeat, Tomato, and Egg Salad Sandwich

*Sliced fillings should be arranged to fit the sandwich. You can always use low-fat mayonnaise instead of the Miracle Whip if you prefer.*

**Yields 4 servings**

Calories: 493
Fat: 14 grams
Protein: 40 grams
Carbohydrates: 55 grams
Cholesterol: 390 milligrams

1½ cups cooked crabmeat
4 tablespoons fat-free Miracle Whip
   salad dressing
12 slices whole wheat bread
2 large tomatoes, thinly sliced
egg salad (page 226)
½ cup coarsely chopped watercress
salt and pepper to taste
1 head of lettuce

1. Smooth crabmeat moistened with a little Miracle Whip on a slice of bread. Top with tomato slices and a dash of salt and pepper to taste. Place another piece of bread over the tomato. Smooth egg salad over the second slice of bread. Top with water cress and finish with the final slice of bread.

# Eggplant and Portobello Mushroom Melt

Extra virgin olive oil can be used instead of canola oil, but it adds
more calories. Use a pastry brush to brush vegetables with oil.

1. Brush the slices of eggplant, onion, and mushroom with the oil. Season with salt and pepper to taste.

2. Grill mushrooms, onion, and eggplant slices on both sides until tender.

3. Mix parsley leaves and thyme with Miracle Whip.

4. Toast or grill individual slices of bread. Thinly spread Miracle Whip mix on grilled side of bread. Arrange slices of vegetables on one side of bread. Top with leaf of lettuce and another slice of grilled bread.

## Sweat Your Eggplant

Eggplant, also known as aubergine, is a member of the nightshade family and is related to tomatoes and potatoes. If eggplant is a little overripe (which happens often with larger eggplant), it will have a bitter taste. To get rid of the bitterness, place the sliced eggplant in a colander and sprinkle with salt. Allow the eggplant to "sweat" for 20 minutes and rinse before using.

**Yields 4 servings**
Calories: 483
Fat: 32 grams
Protein: 9 grams
Carbohydrates: 45 grams
Cholesterol: 3 milligrams

1 large eggplant, sliced lengthwise
    in ½" slices
1 small Vidalia onion, sliced
4 large Portobello mushroom caps
½ cup canola oil
salt and pepper to taste
½ cup fat-free Miracle Whip salad
    dressing
⅓ cup chopped flat-leaf parsley
2 tablespoons fresh thyme
8 slices whole wheat bread
4 leaves lettuce

# Buffalo Mozzarella with Greek Olives and Roasted Red Peppers

Mixing textures enhances flavors—the creaminess of the mozzarella is a nice counterpoint to the salty tang of the olives.

*Yields 12 servings*
Calories: 58
Fat: 1 gram
Protein: 4 grams
Carbohydrates: 11 grams
Cholesterol: 8milligrams

½ cup Greek olives, pitted and
    chopped
½ cup jarred red roasted peppers
    packed in olive oil, chopped
2 tablespoons red wine vinegar
4 ounces buffalo mozzarella, sliced
    thinly
3 large whole wheat pitas

1. Mix the chopped olives and red peppers with the vinegar. Push the mozzarella and vegetables into the pita pockets.

2. Place on a baking sheet. Bake at 350°F until golden brown, about 15 minutes.

3. When browned and hot, cut sandwiches in quarters and serve.

## Buffalo Mozzarella
Unlike most available mozzarella cheese, which is made from cow's milk, buffalo mozzarella is made from the milk of water buffalo. Since buffalo milk contains far more butterfat than cow's milk, the result is a much creamier cheese that is still slightly elastic and mild like other fresh mozzarella cheese.

# Veggie Pitas

This low-calorie, low-fat sandwich is delicious, fresh, and crunchy. Try using other vegetables, too, including bell peppers, summer squash, and mushrooms.

1. Peel cucumber and cut in half. Remove seeds with spoon. Coarsely chop cucumber. Combine with remaining ingredients except pitas and lettuce in medium bowl. Cover and chill for 2 to 3 hours before serving.

2. When ready to serve, heat pitas in toaster oven until warm and pliable. Cut in half and line with lettuce; fill with cucumber mixture. Serve immediately.

## Storing Sandwich Spreads

Any sandwich spread made with mayonnaise, yogurt, or sour cream can be stored, covered, in the refrigerator up to 4 days. Make a couple of these spreads and keep them on hand so your family can make sandwiches or use them as a dip whenever they get hungry.

*Yields 4 servings*
Calories: 134
Fat: 4 grams
Protein: 10 grams
Carbohydrates: 21 grams
Cholesterol: 5 milligrams

1 cucumber
¼ cup chopped scallions
½ cup plain yogurt
¼ cup sour cream
½ teaspoon salt
⅛ teaspoon cayenne pepper
2 carrots, shredded
1 tablespoon fresh oregano leaves
1 cup grape tomatoes, sliced
4 large whole wheat pitas
8 leaves red lettuce

# Monte Cristo Sandwich

**Yields 6–8 servings**
Calories: 373
Fat: 19
Protein: 22 grams
Carbohydrates: 27 grams
Cholesterol: 79 milligrams

*4 slices bacon*
*2 boneless, skinless chicken breasts*
*¼ cup raspberry jam*
*8 slices white bread*
*8 thin slices Gouda cheese*
*4 1-ounce slices ham*
*¼ cup butter, softened*

*Bacon adds a salty crispness to these grilled sandwiches.*
*Serve them with more raspberry jam for dipping.*

1. In medium skillet, cook bacon until crisp. Remove from pan and drain on paper towels; crumble and set aside. Pour drippings from skillet and discard; do not wipe skillet. Add chicken; cook over medium heat, turning once, until browned and cooked, about 8 minutes. Remove chicken from pan and let stand.

2. Spread jam on one side of each slice of bread. Layer half of slices with cheese, then ham. Thinly slice chicken breasts and place over ham. Cover with remaining cheese slices, sprinkle with bacon, and top sandwiches with remaining bread slices.

3. Spread outsides of sandwiches with softened butter. Prepare and preheat griddle, indoor dual-contact grill, or panini maker. Grill sandwiches on medium for 4–6 minutes for dual-contact grill or panini maker, or 6–8 minutes, turning once, for griddle, until bread is golden brown and cheese is melted. Cut in half and serve immediately.

### Sliced Ham

You have several choices when buying sliced ham for sandwiches. You can purchase the super-thin slices packaged in plastic bags, boiled ham in ⅛" slices, or deli ham that you can have sliced to order. Just be sure that the amount of ham you use weighs about 1 ounce per serving to keep the nutrition information constant.

# Ham and Cheese Chutney Sandwich

*Use cooking spray to pan fry this sandwich to keep the calories down.*

1. Coat a pan or griddle with cooking spray over medium heat.

2. Combine Egg Beaters, milk, mustard, cinnamon, salt, and pepper in a medium bowl.

3. Spread chutney on 4 slices of bread. Top with ham and cheese slice and finish with another piece of bread.

4. Place sandwiches in egg mixture and coat on both sides. Cook each sandwich in hot pan, browning on both sides. When cheese is melted, transfer to plates.

*Yields 4 servings*
Calories: 290
Fat: 7 grams
Protein: 22 grams
Carbohydrates: 37 grams
Cholesterol: 20 milligrams

*light cooking spray*
*¼ cup Egg Beaters*
*2 tablespoons fat-free milk*
*1 teaspoon Dijon mustard*
*½ teaspoon cinnamon*
*salt and pepper to taste*
*4 tablespoons prepared mango chutney*
*8 slices whole wheat bread*
*8 slices fat-free baked ham*
*4 slices low-fat Swiss cheese*

# Clubhouse Sandwich

It is easiest to make this club sandwich if you arrange
it on a bread board or a very smooth surface.

**_Yields 4 servings_**
Calories: 513
Fat: 21 grams
Protein: 35 grams
Carbohydrates: 50 grams
Cholesterol: 74 milligrams

_12 slices whole wheat bread_
_3 tablespoons Miracle Whip salad_
_    dressing_
_1 head Romaine lettuce_
_4 large tomatoes, thickly sliced_
_12 slices extra lean bacon, broiled_
_½ pound thinly sliced smoked_
_    turkey_
_salt and pepper to taste_
_12 toothpicks or cocktail sticks_

1.  Toast bread. Spread Miracle Whip thinly on 4 slices of bread. Cut romaine leaves to fit the bread. Place 2 tomato slices next on top of lettuce. Place bacon on top of the tomato. Top with turkey slices, salt, and pepper, and finish with another slice of bread.

2.  Repeat for the second layer. Cover with a final bread slice spread with Miracle Whip.

3.  Cut sandwich into 4 pieces, diagonally. Place toothpick or cocktail stick into center of each little sandwich to hold it together.

## Super Sandwich Sides

In restaurants, this sandwich is typically served with French fries or potato chips. Choose a healthier alternative for your homemade clubhouse sandwiches. This sandwich goes well alongside a small portion of low-fat cottage cheese or some baked chips.

# Conway Welsh Rarebit Melt

Using whole wheat English muffins saves calories. Broil the bacon to get the extra fat off.

1. Melt butter in a saucepan over low heat. Add flour; whisk mixture until smooth.

2. Pour in beer and boil for 3 minutes, continuing to whisk.

3. Reduce heat; add cheddar cheese, Worcestershire sauce, and Tabasco sauce. Continue to cook until all ingredients are combined. Pour mixture over toasted muffins and serve.

## Welsh Rarebit

This sandwich's origins come directly from Conwy, Wales. It's an eighteenth-century dish, served in taverns throughout England, and usually garnished with tomato and parsley.

*Yields 4 servings;*
*serving size 1 melt*
Calories: 365
Fat: 17 grams
Protein: 20 grams
Carbohydrates: 33 grams
Cholesterol: 43 milligrams

¼ cup unsalted butter
¼ cup flour
½ cup light beer
½ pound low-fat extra sharp
   cheddar cheese, grated
2–3 drops Tabasco sauce
½ teaspoon Worcestershire sauce
8 halves whole wheat English
   muffins

# Tuna Melt

*You can use whole wheat bread instead of pita halves.*

**_Yields 4 servings_**
Calories: 535
Fat: 35 grams
Protein: 20 grams
Carbohydrates: 40 grams
Cholesterol: 35 milligrams

1 6-ounce can flaked tuna, packed
    in water
1 small Vidalia onion, finely
    chopped
¼ cup black olives, chopped
½ tomato, finely chopped
2 tablespoons flat-leaf parsley,
    chopped
½ cup olive oil
2 tablespoons cider vinegar
½ cup crumbled feta cheese
4 whole wheat pitas, halved and
    opened

1. Combine tuna, onion, olives, tomato, and parsley in medium bowl. Add oil and vinegar and mix ingredients well.

2. Mound mixture into pita halves and top with feta cheese crumbs.

3. Place under broiler until feta cheese melts.

# Onion and Chicken Sandwich

*You can fry the chicken breasts in any type of oil, but olive and vegetable are recommended.*

1. Combine ground chicken, parsley, onion, hot pepper sauce, and garlic in a medium bowl. Mold into four patties.

2. Heat the olive oil in a large skillet. Place patties in the skillet. Cook patties for 5 minutes on each side.

3. Toast hamburger buns under the broiler. Spread buns with margarine. Serve patties on buttered buns with some chopped parsley.

*Yields 4 servings*
Calories: 383
Fat: 25 grams
Protein: 22 grams
Carbohydrates: 21 grams
Cholesterol: 75 grams

1 pound ground chicken breast
⅓ cup chopped parsley
1 small Vidalia onion, finely chopped
⅓ teaspoon hot pepper sauce
1 teaspoon minced garlic
2 tablespoons olive oil
4 lite hamburger buns, halved
3 tablespoons margarine

# Thanksgiving Wrap

You don't have to wait for Turkey Day leftovers to enjoy these!

1. Toss all but the lettuce together in a large bowl.

2. Lay out the lettuce leaves, add turkey filling, and roll them up.

## Cranberry Additions

Dried cranberries make a tasty addition to many everyday foods. Add them to cereal, trail mix, oatmeal cookies, chocolate chip cookies, and salads for a sweet and tart surprise.

**Yields 12 servings**
Calories: 89
Fat: 3 grams
Protein: 11 grams
Carbohydrates: 3 grams
Cholesterol: 18 milligrams

2 cups cooked turkey, diced
1 stalk celery, minced
½ cup red seedless grapes, halved
2 tablespoons red onion, minced
¼ cup dried cranberries
6 tablespoons low-fat mayonnaise
1 teaspoon dried thyme
salt and pepper to taste
12 large romaine lettuce leaves

# Spicy Ranch Chicken Wrap

*This wrap can be made ahead of time and placed in the refrigerator, tightly covered, until ready to serve.*

1. Mix chicken, garlic, hot pepper, and cumin in a saucepan over medium heat. Cook for 15 minutes until chicken is no longer pink.

2. Stir in flour, chicken broth, milk, sour cream, and salt and pepper, mixing occasionally.

3. Heat oven to 350°F. Warm tortillas in the oven.

4. Wrap chicken mixture in warmed tortillas. Drizzle ranch dressing over tortillas and serve.

*Yields 4 servings*
Calories: 325
Fat: 11 grams
Protein: 26 grams
Carbohydrates: 29 grams
Cholesterol: 65 milligrams

*2 cups diced chicken*
*1 teaspoon minced garlic*
*¼ teaspoon ground red hot pepper*
*⅛ teaspoon ground cumin*
*½ cup flour*
*¾ cup chicken broth*
*½ cup fat-free milk*
*2 tablespoons low-fat sour cream*
*salt and pepper to taste*
*4 6" corn tortillas*
*½ cup light ranch dressing*

# Ginger Peanut Chicken Salad Wrap

*The chow mein vegetables will taste better if they are chilled before use.*

**Yields 4 servings**

Calories: 310
Fat: 16 grams
Protein: 16 grams
Carbohydrates: 24 grams
Cholesterol: 36 milligrams

*1 cup chopped chicken breast*
*¼ cup olive oil*
*1 14-ounce can oriental mixed vegetables, drained*
*⅔ cup Miracle Whip salad dressing*
*2 tablespoons reduced-sodium soy sauce*
*1 teaspoon ground ginger*
*4 6" corn tortillas*

1. Sauté chicken breast in olive oil in a large skillet over medium heat. Add vegetables and sauté until chicken is cooked. Transfer chicken and vegetables to a large bowl. Mix in the Miracle Whip, soy sauce, and ginger.

2. Heat the broiler, and warm the tortillas.

3. Spoon chicken mixture into tortillas. Roll up and serve.

## Rolling Tortillas

Lay the tortilla on a flat surface and place the ingredients on one half of the tortilla so that you can fold it over and roll without ingredients spilling out.

# 19

# Low-Calorie Quick Snacks

# Peanut Butter and Celery

**Yields 2 servings**
Calories: 225
Fat: 17 grams
Protein: 10 grams
Carbohydrates: 11 grams
Cholesterol: 0 milligrams

4 celery stalks
4 tablespoons peanut butter
1 tablespoon bacon bits

Substituting bacon bits for raisins is a twist on the old snacking staple ants on a log.

1. Smooth peanut butter into the celery stalks.

2. Sprinkle with bacon bits.

3. Serve immediately or wrap in wet paper towel and refrigerate for 20 minutes.

## Wrapping Celery

To keep your food moist in the refrigerator, rinse a heavy paper towel in water and gently wring out most of the moisture. Wrap celery stalks with the damp paper towel, and your celery will not dry out.

# Cream Cheese and Celery

*Use fat-free, reduced-calorie cream cheese,*
*preferably already whipped to save you time and calories!*

1. Wash and dry celery and leave tips on stalks.

2. Combine the rest of the ingredients in a bowl.

3. Fill each celery stalk to the brim with the cream cheese mixture.

4. Serve immediately or wrap in moistened paper towels and refrigerate.

*Yields 2 servings*

Calories: 55
Fat: 2 grams
Protein: 3 grams
Carbohydrates: 6 grams
Cholesterol: 3 milligrams

*4 stalks celery*
*2 tablespoons fat-free cream cheese*
*2 teaspoons fat-free Miracle Whip*
*    salad dressing*
*2 chopped olives*
*1 teaspoon crushed walnuts*

# Roasted Chickpeas with Parmesan

**Yields 2 servings**
Calories: 100
Fat: 3 grams
Protein: 6 grams
Carbohydrates: 14 grams
Cholesterol: 5 milligrams

½ cup canned chickpeas, drained
2 tablespoons freshly grated
    Parmesan cheese
few drops hot sauce

This spread can be served hot or cold. Omit the hot sauce altogether if you have mild taste buds.

1. Mash chickpeas with fork in a small bowl or mix in a blender until smooth.

2. Mix Parmesan cheese with chickpea mixture.

3. Add hot sauce and blend well. Serve with pita bread crisps.

## Roasted Chickpeas

Roasted chickpeas make a tasty snack on their own. They come in many flavors, and they are good sources of iron, calcium, antioxidants, and protein. They have less fat than peanuts, but be careful to buy low-sodium chickpeas to avoid excess salt.

# Apple with Yogurt and Cinnamon

You can use any other kind of apples, but Granny Smith apples have a tart taste that goes well with the yogurt. Use vanilla-flavored nonfat yogurt for an additional full-tasting treat.

1. Wash, peel, and cut up apple in small pieces.

2. Mix the yogurt, Splenda, and cinnamon in a small bowl. Mix in apple slices.

3. Chill for 20 minutes and serve.

**_Yields 1 serving_**
Calories: 170
Fat: 0 grams
Protein: 6 grams
Carbohydrates: 41 grams
Cholesterol: 5 milligrams

_1 apple_
_½ cup plain nonfat yogurt_
_2 teaspoons Splenda_
_½ teaspoon cinnamon_

# Apple Jell-O Cups

You can use cranberry or lemon Jell-O instead of lime; any flavor will taste fantastic.

*Yields 2 servings*
Calories: 235
Fat: 1 gram
Protein: 18 grams
Carbohydrates: 16 grams
Cholesterol: 0 milligrams

*1 3-ounce package sugar-free lime Jell-O*
*1 apple*
*2 tablespoons light Cool Whip topping*

1.  Make Jell-O according to directions and refrigerate.

2.  Peel and chop apple into small pieces.

3.  When Jell-O is slightly thickened, remove, and add chopped apple. Refrigerate again until firm.

4.  Serve each cup of Jell-O topped with 1 tablespoon whipped topping.

## Cool Whip

Cool Whip was invented by Kraft Foods and introduced in grocery stores nationwide in 1964. It is a non-dairy dessert topping made with coconut oil and palm oil. It now comes in three varieties, Lite, Free, and Sugar Free.

# Rolled Chipped Beef with No-Fat Cream Cheese

*This is a great canapé for parties. Just multiply the amount by
the number of guests and cover and refrigerate until served.*

1. Spread chipped beef slices on pastry board or flat surface.

2. Mix garlic or onion with cream cheese in a small bowl.

3. Spread each beef slice with a thin layer of cream cheese mixture.

4. Carefully roll up beef slices to form a cigar.

5. Secure each beef slice with a toothpick and refrigerate.

*Yields 2 servings*
Calories: 120
Fat: 5 grams
Protein: 10 grams
Carbohydrates: 8 grams
Cholesterol: 10 milligrams

*4 1-ounce slices thinly cut chipped
beef*
*⅓ cup fat-free cream cheese at
room temperature*
*1 tablespoon minced onion or garlic*

# Broiled Chicken Livers

Maple-flavored bacon imparts a different flavor to the chicken livers.

**Yields 2 servings**
Calories: 145
Fat: 7 grams
Protein: 19 grams
Carbohydrates: 1 gram
Cholesterol: 400 milligrams

1 cup cooked chicken livers
salt and pepper to taste
2 slices very lean low-sodium bacon

1. Drain cooked livers and dry.

2. Season with salt and pepper to taste.

3. Wrap a piece of bacon around each liver and secure with a toothpick.

4. Broil until bacon is crisp.

## Broiling Chicken Livers
Before placing chicken livers on the broiler, soak them in any flavor diet soda for about 2 hours. This may sound odd, but they will taste wonderful and your guests will never be able to figure out why they taste so good.

# Pineapple Chunks in Cream Cheese

*You can use fresh strawberries instead of pineapple chunks for a sweeter, less tangy treat.*

1. Dry pineapple chunks lightly with paper towel.

2. Carefully spread cream cheese over each pineapple chunk.

3. Roll each chunk in the chopped mint.

4. Refrigerate for 20 minutes and serve.

*Yields 4 servings*
Calories: 58
Fat: <1 gram
Protein: 5 grams
Carbohydrates: 9 grams
Cholesterol: 3 milligrams

*1 cup canned pineapple chunks in
    water, drained
½ cup fat-free cream cheese,
    softened
⅓ cup finely chopped mint*

# Savory Dill Franks

**Yields 4 servings**
Calories: 233
Fat: 18 grams
Protein: 11 grams
Carbohydrates: 8 grams
Cholesterol: 46 milligrams

*1 12-ounce package mini-sausages, rinsed and drained*
*2 tablespoons spicy brown mustard*
*2 tablespoons relish*
*1 tablespoon fat-free Miracle Whip*

*You can put a few drops of hot sauce into mixture to add more spice.*

1. Mix mustard, relish, and Miracle Whip in a small bowl.

2. Dip each frank into mixture with a toothpick.

3. Drain on a paper towel. Refrigerate for 20 minutes.

## Serving Franks

These franks are also great served cold. They will keep nicely if you prepare them the day before serving and refrigerate them overnight.

# Nutty Orange

If you like your almonds warm, heat them up in the microwave for 10–20 seconds. You can also toast them in a frying pan over low heat. Do not use any oils or butter; place the nuts in the pan dry and toss as you toast so they don't burn.

1. Peel the oranges and separate the sections.
2. Place orange sections on a plate and sprinkle almond halves on top.

*Yields 2 servings*

Calories: 155
Fat: 6 grams
Protein: 5 grams
Carbohydrates: 24 grams
Cholesterol: 0 milligrams

*2 oranges*
*¼ cup almond halves*

# Seasoned Popcorn

**Yields 2 servings**
Calories: 40
Fat: <1 gram
Protein: 1 gram
Carbohydrates: 8 grams
Cholesterol: 0 milligrams

2½ cups unbuttered popcorn
2 tablespoons Mrs. Dash garlic and
herb seasoning

Create your own seasoning by mixing some of your
favorite spices, herbs, or flavorings in a small bowl.

1. In a medium bowl, sprinkle seasoning over popcorn and toss lightly.

## Unbuttered Popcorn

You can find microwaveable unbuttered popcorn in the grocery store or pop it yourself with a good air popper. To avoid unnecessary fats, do not pop the popcorn on a burner with oil or butter. The seasoning will stick to the popcorn and give you all the flavor you need.

# Skinny Baked Potato

*If you like it spicy, mix a dash of Tabasco with salsa before serving over the baked potato.*

1. Prick the potato several times with a fork, then place on a plate.

2. Bake potato in microwave for about five minutes on each side until soft.

3. Cut potato in half lengthwise and place 1 tablespoon of sour cream on each half.

4. Top with the salsa.

*Yields 1 serving*
Calories: 190
Fat: 1 gram
Protein: 7 grams
Carbohydrates: 42 grams
Cholesterol: 5 milligrams

*1 small baked potato*
*½ cup salsa*
*2 tablespoons fat-free sour cream*

# Sesame Corn Wafers

These little wafers are a lot like commercial corn chips,
but they're coated with sesame seeds for more flavor and crunch.

**Yields 16 servings**
Calories: 89
Fat: 7 grams
Protein: 2 grams
Carbohydrates: 7 grams
Cholesterol: 2 milligrams

1 cup masa harina
2 tablespoons white cornmeal
1 teaspoon salt
½ cup boiling water
1 tablespoon butter
½ cup sesame seeds
2 cups canola oil
more salt, if desired

1. Combine masa harina, cornmeal, and salt in large bowl. Add boiling water and butter and stir until a soft dough forms. You may need to add another tablespoon or so of boiling water. Divide dough into 5 equal pieces. Roll out each piece to ⅛" thickness, about a 6"× 6" rectangle, between two sheets of plastic wrap. Remove the top sheet of plastic wrap, sprinkle with some of the sesame seeds and press seeds into the dough. Cut the dough into 1" × ½" pieces. Repeat with remaining dough.

2. Place oil in heavy saucepan and heat over medium high heat to 375°F. Fry chips, about a fourth at a time, until light golden brown. Remove to paper towels, sprinkle with salt, and let cool. Store covered in airtight container.

3. These can also be baked. Add another 1½ to 2 cups of boiling water to the masa harina mixture to make a batter. Drop by teaspoonfuls onto Silpat-lined cookie sheets and sprinkle with sesame seeds. Bake at 450°F for 11–14 minutes or until chips are golden brown.

## Masa Harina

Masa harina is not cornmeal; it is corn flour. You can find it in the ethnic foods aisle of most supermarkets and in Mexican and Hispanic markets. It is very finely ground so the dough will hold together. There is no gluten in corn flour, so you can reroll scraps as long as you want to; they won't get tough.

# 20

# Desserts

# Low-Fat Ice Cream

*Yields 12 servings;*
*serving size 1 scoop*
Calories: 349
Fat: <1 gram
Protein: 14 grams
Carbohydrates: 73 grams
Cholesterol: 8 milligrams

*3 quarts fat-free milk*
*1-ounce box plain gelatin*
*3 cups sugar*
*2 7.5-ounce cans low-fat*
   *evaporated milk*
*3 tablespoons vanilla*

This is a fast homemade ice cream. You can top it with any fresh fruit of your choice.

1. In a medium pot, bring 2 cups of the fat-free milk to a boil.

2. Add the gelatin to the boiling milk.

3. Mix in the sugar and stir until dissolved.

4. Remove from heat and cool.

5. Once cool, add the evaporated milk, the remaining fat-free milk, and the vanilla.

6. Transfer ingredients to a large plastic container and freeze 6 hours before serving.

# Fruit Popsicles

If you do not have an ice crusher, place the ice in a plastic bag and smash it with a hammer or other hard object to crush it before adding it to a blender. The ice is important for bulking up the mixture.

1. Place fruit, juice, and ice in a blender, in that order.

2. Blend on high.

3. Pour ingredients into popsicle molds.

4. Freeze for 1 hour. Remove popsicles from the freezer and insert a popsicle stick into the center of each treat. Return to the freezer and let solidify for another 7–9 hours before eating.

## Homemade Popsicles

If you don't have a popsicle mold, don't fret. Just use paper cups! Allow the popsicles to freeze about 1 hour, then insert popsicle sticks just as you would in the original recipe. If you don't have popsicle sticks, try plastic spoons. Anything that stays in the center of the popsicle and makes a decent handle will work.

_**Yields 6 servings;**_
_**serving size 1 popsicle**_
Calories: 55
Fat: <1 gram
Protein: 1 gram
Carbohydrates: 14 grams
Cholesterol: 0 milligrams

_1 12-ounce bag frozen strawberries_
_3 cups 100% fruit strawberry juice_
_1 cup crushed ice_

# Chocolate Cake

*Yields 12 servings;*
*serving size 1 slice*
Calories: 203
Fat: 3 grams
Protein: 4 grams
Carbohydrates: 42 grams
Cholesterol: <1 milligram

*light cooking spray*
*2 cups all-purpose flour*
*⅓ cup unsweetened cocoa powder*
*1 teaspoon baking soda*
*½ teaspoon salt*
*1 cup sugar*
*2 tablespoons canola oil*
*1 egg white*
*1 cup nonfat vanilla yogurt*
*2 teaspoons vanilla*
*¼ cup fat-free fudge topping or*
*    chocolate syrup*

You can lightly dust this cake with powdered sugar or even cinnamon rather than frosting it.

1. Preheat oven to 350°F.

2. Spray 8" square pan with light cooking spray. Set aside.

3. In a large bowl, mix the flour, cocoa, baking soda, salt, and sugar well.

4. In a medium bowl, thoroughly mix the oil, egg white, yogurt, vanilla, and fudge topping.

5. Add the wet mixture to the dry mixture and mix thoroughly.

6. Pour the batter into the baking pan. Bake for 35 minutes.

# Cheesecake

Pour a little chocolate syrup over each slice to add a little sweet chocolate for a topping.

1. Preheat oven to 350°F.

2. Stir the graham cracker crumbs and butter together until they are evenly mixed.

3. Press crumb mixture into the bottom of a baking pan.

4. Mix cream cheese, Splenda, vanilla, and egg whites in a medium bowl with an electric mixer.

5. Add the cake flour, salt, and milk. Mix thoroughly.

6. Pour batter into the crust. Bake for 1 hour.

7. Cool before placing in fridge.

8. Refrigerate at least 3 hours before serving.

## Freezing Cheesecake

To safely freeze a cheesecake, place it in the freezer uncovered until it is frozen through. Tightly wrap the cheesecake in two layers of plastic wrap and cover with aluminum foil. Do not keep the cheesecake frozen for longer than a month. When you are ready to eat the cheesecake, thaw it out by removing it to the refrigerator overnight.

_Yields 8 servings_
Calories: 246
Fat: 8 grams
Protein: 12 grams
Carbohydrates: 31 grams
Cholesterol: 20 milligrams

1 cup reduced-fat graham crackers, finely crushed
¼ cup butter, melted
16 ounces fat-free cream cheese
½ cup Splenda
1 teaspoon vanilla
2 egg whites
3 tablespoons cake flour
¼ teaspoon salt
½ cup fat-free milk

# Mama's Cupcakes

**Yields 12 servings**
Calories: 121
Fat: <1 gram
Protein: 6 grams
Carbohydrates: 23 grams
Cholesterol: 0 milligrams

1 cup self-rising flour
½ cup nonfat dried milk powder
1 3.4-ounce box sugar-free
    chocolate Jell-O pudding mix
1 tablespoon unsweetened cocoa
½ cup Splenda
1 teaspoon vanilla
½ cup applesauce
¼ teaspoon baking soda
4 egg whites
pinch of salt

To see if your cupcakes are done, insert a clean toothpick into the center of a cupcake. The toothpick should come out clean. You can also tell by gently pressing on the top of the cupcake with a spoon; if the cupcake bounces back with spring, the batch is done.

1. Preheat oven to 350°F.

2. Mix flour, milk powder, Jell-O mix, cocoa, and Splenda in a medium bowl.

3. In a separate bowl, blend the vanilla, applesauce, and baking soda.

4. In a small bowl, beat the egg whites and salt until stiff.

5. Add the flour mixture to the egg whites, beating with an electric mixer.

6. Add the applesauce and beat until blended.

7. Line a muffin tin with paper cupcake wrappers and fill each ¾ of the way with batter.

8. Bake for 20 minutes.

# Banana Nut Cake

*You can drizzle honey over each slice of cake to add some scrumptious sweetness.*

1. Preheat oven to 350°F.

2. Lightly spray a 9" x 13" cooking pan and set aside.

3. In a large mixing bowl, combine the cake mix and walnuts.

4. Add the milk, bananas, Egg Beaters, and oil, and mix well.

5. Spread batter into baking pan.

6. Bake for 30 minutes or until browned on top.

## Overripe Bananas

Overripe bananas work best for this recipe because they are easier to mash. If you have way too many overripe bananas, refrigerate them to keep the flesh firm and use them in banana baking recipes. They also make fantastic additions to any shake or smoothie.

*Yields 16 servings*
Calories: 199
Fat: 4 grams
Protein: 4 grams
Carbohydrates: 30 grams
Cholesterol: 1 milligram

*light cooking spray*
*1 18-ounce box yellow cake mix*
*½ cup chopped walnuts*
*1 cup fat-free milk*
*1 cup mashed bananas*
*1 cup Egg Beaters*
*1 tablespoon olive oil*

# Chocolate Layer Cake

Frost this cake with sugar-free Cool Whip and serve immediately.

**_Yields 24 servings_**
Calories: 84
Fat: 4 grams
Protein: 2 grams
Carbohydrates: 11 grams
Cholesterol: 11 milligrams

_light cooking spray_
_1 cup hot water_
_⅔ cup unsweetened cocoa powder_
_1¾ cup Splenda_
_1 stick of butter_
_2 teaspoons vanilla_
_3 egg whites_
_½ cup fat-free sour cream_
_1¾ cups cake flour_
_1 teaspoon baking powder_
_½ teaspoon baking soda_
_1 teaspoon salt_

1. Preheat oven to 350°F.

2. Spray 9" round cake pans with light cooking spray.

3. Combine hot water and the cocoa powder in a medium bowl.

4. Cream the Splenda and butter in a large bowl with an electric mixer.

5. Mix in the vanilla and egg whites, beating well as you go.

6. Add the sour cream and beat for 2 minutes.

7. In a medium bowl, mix the flour, baking powder, baking soda, and salt.

8. Add the dry mixture to the batter and beat on low speed.

9. Add in the cocoa mixture, beating well.

10. Pour batter into baking pans and bake for 30 minutes or until a toothpick inserted into the center comes out clean.

11. Cool before removing cake from pans.

# Caramel Sour Cream Cake

*Drizzle this cake with some purchased caramel ice cream
topping for a decadent dessert with a minimal amount of calories!*

*Yields 16 servings*
Calories: 140
Fat: 4 grams
Protein: 3 grams
Carbohydrates: 24 grams
Cholesterol: 33 milligrams

1 cup sour cream
½ cup sugar
½ cup brown sugar
2 eggs
2 teaspoons vanilla
1¾ cups flour
1 teaspoon baking powder
1 teaspoon baking soda
¼ teaspoon salt
¼ teaspoon ground nutmeg

1. Preheat oven to 350°F. Grease 9" × 13" pan with unsalted butter and set aside.

2. In a large bowl, combine sour cream and sugar; beat well. Add brown sugar and beat. Add eggs, one at a time, beating well after each addition. Stir in vanilla.

3. Sift flour with baking powder, baking soda, salt, and nutmeg. Stir into sour cream mixture and beat at medium speed for 1 minute. Pour into prepared pan.

4. Bake for 25 to 35 minutes or until cake pulls away from sides of pan and top springs back when lightly touched in center. Cool completely on wire rack; store covered at room temperature.

## What Is Caramel?

Caramel is created when sugar is melted. When sugar is melted and reaches 338°F, the molecules in the sugar begin to break down and recombine to form other compounds. These new compounds create the color and complex, rich flavor of caramel. Brown sugar does not contain caramel; it's regular granulated sugar combined with molasses.

# Honey Cakes

**Yields 24 servings**
Calories: 187
Fat: 4 grams
Protein: 3 grams
Carbohydrates: 36 grams
Cholesterol: 0 milligrams

3½ cups flour
¼ teaspoon salt
1½ teaspoons baking powder
1 teaspoon baking soda
2 teaspoons ground cinnamon
1½ teaspoons allspice
1¼ cup Egg Beaters
¾ cup Splenda
4 tablespoons vegetable oil
light cooking spray
½ cup almonds
1½ cups honey
2 tablespoons lemon juice
½ cup water

*If you find your honey a little too sticky, heat it in the microwave for 5 seconds to thin it out.*

1. Preheat oven to 325°F.

2. Combine the flour, salt, baking powder, baking soda, cinnamon, and allspice in a large bowl.

3. In a medium bowl, thoroughly mix the Egg Beaters, vegetable oil, and Splenda.

4. Stir into the flour mixture.

5. Chop the almonds coarsely and stir them into the batter.

6. Lightly spray two 9" round baking pans.

7. Fill pans with batter and bake for about 1 hour to 1½ hours or until cakes are done.

8. Let cakes cool.

9. Meanwhile, boil water, honey, and lemon juice until it forms a thick glaze. Drizzle over cake.

# Gingerbread

Sprinkle this cake lightly with a little powdered sugar before serving.

1. In a large bowl, mix the sugar and margarine with an electric mixer until well blended.

2. Add the molasses and egg. Mix well.

3. Mix the flour, ginger, baking soda, nutmeg, cloves, and salt in a large bowl.

4. Add the flour mixture to sugar mixture.

5. Add the milk and mix well.

6. Lightly spray a square baking pan.

7. Pour batter into the pan.

8. Bake for about 30 minutes or until done.

## Sweet Ginger

Queen Elizabeth I may have invented the gingerbread man, but Chinese cooks have been putting ginger's subtle flavor to use since ancient times. Many people serve gingerbread to soothe an upset stomach or nausea, and nothing beats a comforting cup of ginger tea when you're feeling run down.

**Yields 10 servings**
Calories: 196
Fat: 5 grams
Protein: 3 grams
Carbohydrates: 34 grams
Cholesterol: 22 milligrams

⅓ cup sugar
¼ cup margarine
½ cup molasses
1 egg
1½ cups flour
1 teaspoon ground ginger
½ teaspoon baking soda
¼ teaspoon ground nutmeg
⅛ teaspoon ground cloves
⅛ teaspoon salt
⅔ cup fat-free milk
light cooking spray

# Butterscotch Cupcakes

Use butterscotch ice cream topping as the frosting
for these cupcakes, about 1 tablespoon per cupcake.

*Yields 16 servings*

Calories: 82
Fat: <1 gram
Protein: 2 grams
Carbohydrates: 19 grams
Cholesterol: <1 milligram

*½ cup cake flour*
*¾ cup powdered sugar*
*5 egg whites*
*⅛ teaspoon salt*
*1 teaspoon heavy cream*
*½ cup butterscotch ice cream*
  *topping*
*¼ cup granulated sugar*
*½ teaspoon vanilla*

1. Preheat oven to 350°F.

2. Line muffin tins with cupcake liners and set aside.

3. In a large bowl, sift the cake flour and powdered sugar twice.

4. In a medium bowl, beat the egg whites and salt with an electric mixer until frothy.

5. Add heavy cream and butterscotch until soft peaks form.

6. Add sugar and continue beating.

7. Fold in flour mixture gradually until blended.

8. Add vanilla. Mix thoroughly.

9. Spoon batter into muffin cups.

10. Bake for 20 minutes or until cupcake tops are browned.

The Everything Calorie Counting Cookbook

# Applesauce Sour Cream Coffee Cake

*You can also peel an apple and chop up pieces to add to the cake if you like.*

1. Preheat oven to 350°F.

2. Coat a square baking pan with light cooking spray.

3. Mix the flour, brown sugar, baking soda, baking powder, cinnamon, and salt in a large bowl.

4. Mix the sour cream, oil, and applesauce in a small bowl.

5. Add sour cream mixture to flour mixture. Mix well but do not beat.

6. Pour batter into cake pan and bake until done, about 40 minutes.

## Avoiding Caffeine

Coffee cakes are meant to be enjoyed with a steaming mug of coffee, but you should avoid coffee, tea, and soft drinks with caffeine. Caffeine can lower your blood sugar, causing you to crave sugar and sweets. Instead, eat this coffee cake with a glass of fat-free skim milk or one of the delicious smoothies or shakes in Chapter 4.

*Yields 20 servings;*
*serving size 1 slice*
Calories: 92
Fat: 2 grams
Protein: 1 gram
Carbohydrates: 18 grams
Cholesterol: 1 milligram

*light cooking spray*
*1½ cups flour*
*¾ cup packed light brown sugar*
*½ teaspoon baking powder*
*1 teaspoon baking soda*
*1 teaspoon ground cinnamon*
*1 teaspoon salt*
*¾ cup fat-free sour cream*
*2 tablespoons canola oil*
*1 cup unsweetened applesauce*

# Apple Cake

Before you add the apple juice, heat it in the microwave
to warm it. It blends better with the oats this way.

**Yields 10 servings**
Calories: 297
Fat: 13 grams
Protein: 4 grams
Carbohydrates: 43 grams
Cholesterol: 0 milligrams

1 cup uncooked oats
¾ cup apple juice
2 tablespoons canola oil
¼ cup Egg Beaters
2 teaspoons vanilla
1 stick margarine, melted
1 cup packed brown sugar
1 large Granny Smith apple, peeled
   and thinly sliced
1¼ cup flour
1 teaspoon baking soda
1 teaspoon cinnamon
½ teaspoon salt
¼ teaspoon ground nutmeg

1. Mix the oats, juice, and oil in a medium bowl.

2. Add the Egg Beaters and vanilla. Mix thoroughly.

3. Preheat oven to 350°F.

4. Pour melted margarine in the bottom of a 9" cake pan.

5. Sprinkle cake pan with ¼ cup of brown sugar.

6. Arrange apple slices on top of sugar.

7. Mix the remaining brown sugar with the flour, baking soda, cinnamon, salt, and nutmeg in a large bowl. Combine thoroughly.

8. Add the oatmeal mixture, blending well.

9. Add batter to cake pan on top of apple slices.

10. Bake 35–45 minutes or until done.

11. Cool in pan, then place a plate upside down on top of cake and invert it.

# John's Apple Crisp

The key to apple crisp is the oatmeal mixture. You need the brown sugar, margarine, and cinnamon well mixed. If you like more "crisp" to your apple crisp, add more oats and margarine.

1. Preheat oven to 350°F.

2. Combine apples, lemon juice, and sugar in a large bowl, tossing to mix.

3. Place this apple mixture on the bottom of a 9" pie plate.

4. In a medium bowl, mix the oats, Splenda brown sugar, margarine, and cinnamon with your fingers to make sure the mixture is crumbly.

5. Sprinkle crumb mixture over apple mixture.

6. Bake about 50 minutes or until bubbly.

_**Yields 6 servings**_
Calories: 157
Fat: 5 grams
Protein: 2 grams
Carbohydrates: 31 grams
Cholesterol: 0 milligrams

4 Granny Smith apples, peeled and sliced
1 tablespoon lemon juice
3 tablespoons sugar
1 cup uncooked oats
2 tablespoons Splenda brown sugar
2 tablespoons margarine
1 teaspoon ground cinnamon

# Mango Angel Fluff

*This light dessert is delicious served with a raspberry sauce made by puréeing frozen thawed raspberries with a little lemon juice.*

**Yields 12 servings**
Calories: 148
Fat: 6 grams
Protein: 2 grams
Carbohydrates: 24 grams
Cholesterol: 14 milligrams

*4 pasteurized egg whites*
*1 cup sugar*
*1 tablespoon lemon juice*
*7.5 ounces frozen mangoes, thawed*
*1 cup heavy whipping cream*
*2 tablespoons powdered sugar*
*1 teaspoon vanilla*
*1 cup flaked coconut*

1. Place egg whites in a large bowl; let stand for 30 minutes at room temperature. Add sugar, lemon juice, and mangoes. Beat with a hand mixer until combined, then beat for 15 minutes at high speed, until mixture is thick and triples in volume.

2. In a medium bowl, beat cream with powdered sugar and vanilla until stiff. Fold into meringue along with coconut. Rinse a 10-inch ring mold with water and shake out over sink; do not dry mold. Pour coconut mixture into mold. Cover and freeze until firm.

3. To unmold, rinse a kitchen towel in hot water and wring out. Place mold on serving plate. Drape hot towel over mold for 10 to 15 seconds to loosen dessert. Remove mold, let stand at room temperature for 15 minutes, slice, and serve with raspberry sauce.

### Pasteurized Egg Whites

When recipes call for raw eggs, you should consider using pasteurized eggs. They are more expensive but worth it. Be sure to watch the expiration date on these eggs and discard them after that date has passed. It does take longer for pasteurized whites to whip, but just keep working; they will fluff up.

# Lemon Pie

*Lemon zest is the grated rind of the lemon. Gather the zest before you squeeze the lemon for the juice. Use a zester to scrape off the yellow skin. Do not zest the bitter white underskin.*

1. Squeeze the lemons to get ½ cup of juice.

2. In a double boiler, cook the Egg Beaters, sugar, and lemon juice over simmering water until it gets thick.

3. Remove from heat and stir in the lemon zest.

4. Pour entire mixture into a medium bowl and stick in refrigerator until it is cold.

5. Whip the egg whites to form stiff peaks.

6. Mix about ⅓ of the egg whites into the cold lemon mixture.

7. Fold in the rest of the whites and the Cool Whip topping until it is all well blended.

8. Crush the vanilla wafers in a freezer bag.

9. Line 2 pie tins with vanilla wafer crumbs, saving some to sprinkle over the tops of the pies.

10. Fill the pie tins with the lemon mixture. Sprinkle the remaining crumbs over the tops. Place the pies in the freezer until firm.

11. Remove from the freezer about 10 minutes before you plan to serve to slightly thaw and make it easier to slice.

*Yields 12 servings*
Calories: 155
Fat: 5 grams
Protein: 3 grams
Carbohydrates: 24 grams
Cholesterol: 7 milligrams

*zest and juice of 2 lemons*
*½ cup Egg Beaters*
*½ cup sugar*
*4 pasteurized egg whites*
*4 cups light Cool Whip*
*5½ ounces vanilla wafer cookies*

# Pumpkin Pie

If you prefer a smooth crust, roll the dough into a circle
and press it out to about 11" and then drape into the pie pan.

**Yields 12 servings**
Calories: 182
Fat: 6 grams
Protein: 4 grams
Carbohydrates: 28 grams
Cholesterol: 26 milligrams

¾ cup packed brown sugar
¼ teaspoon salt
2 teaspoons cinnamon
1 tablespoon nutmeg
12 ounces evaporated low-fat milk
2 egg whites
1 whole egg
15 ounces unsweetened pumpkin
8 ounces packaged pie dough
light cooking spray

1. Preheat oven 425°F.

2. Mix the sugar, salt, cinnamon, nutmeg, evaporated milk, egg whites, whole egg, and pumpkin in a large bowl. Stir with a whisk and set aside.

3. Spray pie pan with the light cooking spray.

4. Press the dough into the pie pan, covering the bottom and all sides.

5. Pour the pie mixture into the pie plate.

6. Bake for 50 minutes.

## Canned Pumpkin

When a recipe calls for canned pumpkin, be sure you buy and use what is called "solid pack" pumpkin. If you use canned pumpkin-pie filling, the recipe will fail because that ingredient contains sugar, emulsifiers, and liquids in addition to pumpkin. If you're feeling ambitious, you could cook and puree a fresh pumpkin and use that.

# Apple Pie

*Make sure the ice water is ice cold; this is the key to making the pie crust.*

1. Combine ½ cup flour, ice water, and vinegar, stirring with a whisk until well blended.

2. Mix in the remaining 1½ cups flour, powdered sugar, and ½ teaspoon salt in a large bowl.

3. Mix in shortening with 2 knives until mixture resembles coarse meal.

4. Divide dough in half.

5. Gently press each half into a 4" circle on 2 sheets of overlapping heavy-duty plastic wrap; cover with 2 additional sheets of overlapping plastic wrap.

6. Roll 1 dough half, still covered, into a 12" circle. Repeat with the other half. Chill dough 10 minutes or until plastic wrap can be easily removed.

7. Prepare filling by combining the apples and lemon juice in a large bowl.

8. Mix ⅔ cup sugar, 3 tablespoons flour, cinnamon, nutmeg, and ⅛ teaspoon salt in a small bowl.

9. Sprinkle sugar mixture over apples and toss well to coat.

10. Lightly spray pie plates with cooking spray.

11. Remove top 2 sheets of plastic wrap from 12" dough circle. Fit dough, plastic wrap side up, into the pie plate, allowing dough to extend over edge.

12. Remove remaining plastic wrap. Spoon filling into dough; brush edges of dough lightly with water.

13. Remove top 2 sheets of plastic wrap from the remaining dough circle; place, plastic wrap side up, on top of filled pie plate. Remove remaining plastic wrap. Press edges of dough together. Fold edges under. Cut several 1" slits in top of pastry using a sharp knife.

14. Brush top and edges of pie with egg white; sprinkle with 1 tablespoon sugar.

15. Bake for 40 minutes or until top is golden brown. Chill well before serving.

*Yields 10 servings*
Calories: 285
Fat: 9 grams
Protein: 3 grams
Carbohydrates: 50 grams
Cholesterol: 0 milligrams

*2 cups all-purpose flour, divided*
*6 tablespoons ice water*
*1 teaspoon cider vinegar*
*2 tablespoons powdered sugar*
*½ teaspoon salt*
*7 tablespoons vegetable shortening*
*8 cups Granny Smith apples, peeled and thinly sliced*
*1 tablespoon fresh lemon juice*
*⅔ cup sugar*
*3 tablespoons all-purpose flour*
*1 teaspoon cinnamon*
*1 teaspoon ground nutmeg*
*1 teaspoon salt*
*1 egg white*
*1 tablespoon sugar*

# Chocolate Chip Peanut Butter Pie

**Yields 10 servings**
Calories: 319
Fat: 14 grams
Protein: 7 grams
Carbohydrates: 43 grams
Cholesterol: 1 milligram

2 14-ounce packages fat-free
    chocolate pudding
½ cup smooth reduced-fat peanut
    butter
1 9" graham cracker crust
1 8-ounce container low-fat
    whipped topping

Folding ingredients means you want to blend them together
but not mix them completely. With this recipe it creates layers of flavor.

1. Fold the pudding and peanut butter together in a large bowl.

2. Pour filling into pie crust and freeze until firm.

3. Thaw in refrigerator for 2 hours before serving.

4. Top with low-fat whipped topping before serving.

## Pie Toppings

You can melt a handful of chocolate chips or peanut butter chips and drizzle them over the top of the pie or decorate the pie with Reese's cups cut in half. You can also freeze it with these toppings to add flavor layers.

# Frozen Yogurt Pie

*You can make this pie in any flavor. Just change the flavor of the yogurt and gelatin.*

1. Mix the strawberries and yogurt in a blender or food processor and blend until mostly creamy with small chunks of strawberries.

2. Mix the whipped topping and gelatin in a large bowl.

3. Mix in the strawberry/yogurt mixture.

4. Pour the mixture into the baked pastry shell and freeze.

5. Serve frozen or partially thawed.

*Yields 10 servings*
Calories: 186
Fat: 4 grams
Protein: 4 grams
Carbohydrates: 29 grams
Cholesterol: <1 milligram

*1 16-ounce package frozen strawberries, defrosted*
*2 8-ounce containers nonfat vanilla yogurt*
*1 8-ounce container low-fat or nonfat frozen whipped topping*
*1 2-ounce package strawberry gelatin*
*1 9" pre-baked pie shell*

# Peach Pie

_**Yields 10 servings**_
Calories: 190
Fat: 4 grams
Protein: 2 grams
Carbohydrates: 37 grams
Cholesterol: 0 milligrams

_1 3-ounce package sugar-free
    peach Jell-O_
_1 cup Splenda_
_2 tablespoons cornstarch_
_1 9" pre-baked pie crust_
_1 8-ounce can sliced peaches_
_1 cup water_

_Instead of canned peaches, peel and slice your own. Top this pie with low-fat Cool Whip._

1.  Mix the dry Jell-O, Splenda, cornstarch, and water in a pot and bring to a boil for 3 minutes, then cool.

2.  Arrange peaches in the pie shell.

3.  Pour Jell-O mixture over peaches and refrigerate.

### Canned vs. Fresh Fruit

Pies are one of the few sweets for which canned fruits can be easily substituted for fresh fruits. Such desserts are particularly welcome during the cold winter months. Just be sure to drain the fruit thoroughly before using it in the recipe. Otherwise you could end up with mush.

# Classic Oatmeal Cookies

*Add a cup of raisins or ½ cup of pecans if you like.*

1. Preheat oven to 375°F.

2. Prepare baking sheets with light cooking spray. Set aside.

3. Beat the sugar and margarine in a large bowl with a hand mixer.

4. Add the eggs, applesauce, and vanilla, mixing well.

5. Combine flour, baking soda, and salt in a medium bowl.

6. Add flour mixture to sugar mixture. Beat well.

7. Stir in the oats and mix well.

8. Drop dough into mounds on baking sheets, about 2 inches apart.

9. Bake 15 minutes or until cookies are golden brown.

*Yields 24 cookies*
Calories: 218
Fat: 5 grams
Protein: 4 grams
Carbohydrates: 39 grams
Cholesterol: 35 milligrams

1 cup sugar
¼ cup margarine, softened
2 eggs
¾ cup unsweetened applesauce
1 teaspoon vanilla
2 cups flour
½ teaspoon baking soda
¼ teaspoon salt
1 cup uncooked oats
light cooking spray

# Ginger Cookies

*Ginger cookies are done when the tops start to crack in the oven.*
*Once you see the cracking, pull them out and let them harden.*

**Yields 20 cookies**
Calories: 138
Fat: 4 grams
Protein: 2 grams
Carbohydrates: 24 grams
Cholesterol: 0 milligrams

1¼ cup flour
2 teaspoons ground ginger
¼ cup packed brown sugar
¼ teaspoon vanilla
¼ cup molasses
3 tablespoons margarine, melted
1 egg white, lightly beaten
¼ cup unsweetened applesauce
light cooking spray

1. Sift flour and ginger in a large bowl, then stir in sugar.

2. Mix the vanilla, molasses, margarine, applesauce, and egg white in a medium bowl.

3. Add wet ingredients to the dry and stir until well blended.

4. Place dough in freezer until firm.

5. Preheat oven to 350°F.

6. Shape firm dough into balls and drop onto a baking sheet.

7. Bake 12 minutes and let cool.

## Chilling Cookie Dough

Cookie dough is usually chilled before use to make it easier to handle. But chilling dough has other advantages. It lets you use a bit less flour, which results in a more tender cookie. And it lets the gluten in the flour relax, so the dough is easier to handle and rolls without springing back.

# Sugar Cookies

*If you like sugar cookies with extra flavor, add orange extract
for a very vanilla-and-orange-flavored sugar cookie.*

1. Preheat oven to 350°F.

2. Mix all dry ingredients in a large bowl.

3. Mix all liquid ingredients in a medium bowl; add to dry ingredients and mix thoroughly.

4. Spray baking sheets with light spray.

5. Drop cookie dough balls about 2 inches apart on baking sheet.

6. Bake 8–10 minutes or until slightly browned on edges.

**_Yields 20 cookies_**
Calories: 172
Fat: 5 grams
Protein: 3 grams
Carbohydrates: 29 grams
Cholesterol: 21 milligrams

*1 cup flour*
*½ cup whole wheat flour*
*¾ cup sugar*
*¼ teaspoon salt*
*1 teaspoon baking powder*
*3 tablespoons canola oil*
*1 egg*
*2 tablespoons skim milk*
*2 teaspoons vanilla*
*light cooking spray*

# Crisp Icebox Cookies

You can substitute any nut you'd like in these delicious little crisp cookies.
Finely chopped macadamia nuts would be an excellent choice.

***Yields 48 cookies***
Calories: 118
Fat: 6 grams
Protein: 1 gram
Carbohydrates: 15 grams
Cholesterol: 16 milligrams

*¾ cup butter, softened*
*¼ cup coconut oil*
*1 cup brown sugar*
*1 cup sugar*
*2 eggs*
*2 teaspoons vanilla*
*2¼ cups flour*
*1 teaspoon baking soda*
*½ teaspoon salt*
*1 cup finely chopped cashews*

1. In a large bowl, beat butter and coconut oil until blended. Gradually add brown sugar and sugar; beat until fluffy. Add eggs and vanilla and mix well. Stir in flour, baking soda, and salt.

2. Shape dough into 3 long rolls, about 1½" in diameter. Roll the cookie rolls in the chopped cashews, gently pressing nuts into dough to adhere. Wrap well in wax paper, then put rolls into plastic food-storage bags. Chill for at least 24 hours.

3. Preheat oven to 375°F. Cut the dough into slices about ¼" thick and place on ungreased baking sheets. Bake for 6 to 8 minutes or until cookies are very light golden brown and set. Cool on cookie sheets for 3 minutes, then remove to wire racks to cool.

## Icebox Cookies

If you're pressed for time, icebox cookies are a great choice. You can make the dough one day, then chill it in the refrigerator and bake the next day, or the next. These cookie doughs also freeze very well. Wrap them in freezer wrap and place them in freezer plastic bags. You can slice and bake the dough frozen; just add a few minutes to the baking time.

The Everything Calorie Counting Cookbook

# A

## Suggested Menus

When planning out your menus, remember to be creative and have fun. Think in terms of food tastes and textures. Don't deprive yourself of dessert, but build it into your calorie counting so that you have the fun of always having dessert instead of only when you think you can. This way, every meal will be a treat worth working for.

## Family Dinner
Cheese Straws
Dilled Tomato and Onion Salad
Tuna Burgers
Applesauce Sour Cream Coffee Cake

## Dinner for Two
Grilled Herbed Tomatoes
Lime-Seared Scallops
Grilled Artichokes
Chocolate Layer Cake

## Sunday Brunch
Stuffed French Toast
Strawberry Smoothies
Classic Oatmeal Cookies

## Picnic on the Lawn
Cherry-Berry Scones
Pear and Watercress Salad
Mama's Egg Salad Sandwich
Banana Nut Cake

## Holiday Dinner
Crunchy Party Mix
French Onion Soup
Orange Cracked-Wheat Bread
Simple Tomato and Mozzarella Salad
Flank Steak
John's Apple Crisp

## The-Neighbors-Are-Dropping-By Dinner
Chunky Vegetable Dip
Apricot Muffins
Mary's Marvelous Marinated Mushrooms

Crab and Corn Pasta
Butterscotch Cupcakes

## You're-On-the-Go-All-Day Meals
Breakfast Smoothie (any type)
Cranberry Muffin
Gazpacho
Sinfully Thin Salad
Bacon, Lettuce, and Tomato Sandwich
Apple and Yogurt with Cinnamon
Fruit Popsicle

## Birthday Dinner
Light and Little Pizzas
Cucumber and Red Onion Salad
Creamy Cheese and Buttermilk Dressing
Pulled Chicken BBQ
Chocolate Layer Cake

## Fun-with-Friends Cookout
Cheese, Olive, and Cherry Tomato Kabobs
Grilled Tuna with Vegetables
Tartar Sauce
Grilled Artichokes
Salmon Salad
Lemon and Oil Dressing
Honey Cakes

## Take Your Lunch to Work
Oatmeal Banana Bread
Clubhouse Sandwich
Roasted Chickpeas with Parmesan

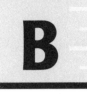

# B

# Resources

## Web Sites

### My Food Diary Calorie Counter

*www.myfooddiary.com*

This Web site provides tools to track calories and eating habits for sustained weight loss and control as well as a healthier overall diet.

### The Calorie Counter

*www.thecaloriecounter.com*

Another online calorie-counting resource.

### USDA Food Pyramid

*www.mypyramid.gov*

The Pyramid, updated in 2005, recommends basing your diet on whole grains, fruits, and vegetables, with moderate exercise.

### USDA My Pyramid Tracker

*www.mypyramidtracker.gov*

My Pyramid Tracker is an online dietary and physical activity tool.

### USDA Calorie Counter Database

*www.breadwithoutborders.com/calorie.htm*

The USDA's searchable database for calorie and nutritional information.

### FDA Information about Losing Weight and Maintaining a Healthy Weight

*www.cfsan.fda.gov/~dms/wh-wght.html*

The Federal Food & Drug Administration's online linking resource for weight loss and weight maintenance with links to numerous other related projects by other federal agencies.

### The American Diabetes Association

*www.diabetes.org/home.jsp*

The American Diabetes Association is a font of information regarding diets and calorie-counting tips.

## Books

Borushek, Allen. *The Calorie King Food & Exercise Journal.* (Costa Mesa, California: Family Health Publications, 2006).

Carpender, Dana. *Dana Carpender's Carb Gram Counte.r* (Gloucester, Massachusetts: Fair Winds Press, 2004).

Holzmeister, Lea Ann. *The Ultimate Calorie, Carb and Fat Gram Counter.* (Alexandria, Virginia: American Diabetes Association, 2006).

Netzer, Corrine T. *The Complete Book of Food Counts.* (New York: Dell Publishing, 2005).

Schaar, Helena. *Fast and EZ Calorie, Fat, Carb, Fiber & Protein Counter.* (Morrisville, North Carolina: Lulu.com, 2004).

Warshaw, Hope L., and the Staff of the American Diabetes Association. *Guide to Healthy Restaurant Eating.* (Alexandria, Virginia: American Diabetes Association, 2005).

Warshaw, Hope L., and Karmeen Kulkari. *Complete Guide to Carb Counting.* (Alexandria, Virginia: American Diabetes Association, 2004).

# Index

# THE EVERYTHING SERIES!

## BUSINESS & PERSONAL FINANCE

Everything® Accounting Book
Everything® Budgeting Book
Everything® Business Planning Book
**Everything® Coaching and Mentoring Book, 2nd Ed.**
Everything® Fundraising Book
Everything® Get Out of Debt Book
Everything® Grant Writing Book
**Everything® Guide to Foreclosures**
Everything® Guide to Personal Finance for Single Mothers
Everything® Home-Based Business Book, 2nd Ed.
Everything® Homebuying Book, 2nd Ed.
Everything® Homeselling Book, 2nd Ed.
Everything® Improve Your Credit Book
Everything® Investing Book, 2nd Ed.
Everything® Landlording Book
Everything® Leadership Book
Everything® Managing People Book, 2nd Ed.
Everything® Negotiating Book
Everything® Online Auctions Book
Everything® Online Business Book
Everything® Personal Finance Book
Everything® Personal Finance in Your 20s and 30s Book
Everything® Project Management Book
Everything® Real Estate Investing Book
Everything® Retirement Planning Book
Everything® Robert's Rules Book, $7.95
Everything® Selling Book
Everything® Start Your Own Business Book, 2nd Ed.
Everything® Wills & Estate Planning Book

## COOKING

Everything® Barbecue Cookbook
**Everything® Bartender's Book, 2nd Ed., $9.95**
**Everything® Calorie Counting Cookbook**
Everything® Cheese Book
Everything® Chinese Cookbook
Everything® Classic Recipes Book
Everything® Cocktail Parties & Drinks Book
Everything® College Cookbook
Everything® Cooking for Baby and Toddler Book
Everything® Cooking for Two Cookbook
Everything® Diabetes Cookbook
Everything® Easy Gourmet Cookbook
Everything® Fondue Cookbook
Everything® Fondue Party Book
Everything® Gluten-Free Cookbook
Everything® Glycemic Index Cookbook
Everything® Grilling Cookbook
Everything® Healthy Meals in Minutes Cookbook
Everything® Holiday Cookbook

Everything® Indian Cookbook
Everything® Italian Cookbook
Everything® Low-Carb Cookbook
**Everything® Low-Cholesterol Cookbook**
Everything® Low-Fat High-Flavor Cookbook
Everything® Low-Salt Cookbook
Everything® Meals for a Month Cookbook
Everything® Mediterranean Cookbook
Everything® Mexican Cookbook
Everything® No Trans Fat Cookbook
Everything® One-Pot Cookbook
Everything® Pizza Cookbook
Everything® Quick and Easy 30-Minute,
    5-Ingredient Cookbook
Everything® Quick Meals Cookbook
Everything® Slow Cooker Cookbook
Everything® Slow Cooking for a Crowd Cookbook
Everything® Soup Cookbook
Everything® Stir-Fry Cookbook
**Everything® Sugar-Free Cookbook**
**Everything® Tapas and Small Plates Cookbook**
Everything® Tex-Mex Cookbook
Everything® Thai Cookbook
Everything® Vegetarian Cookbook
Everything® Wild Game Cookbook
Everything® Wine Book, 2nd Ed.

## GAMES

Everything® 15-Minute Sudoku Book, $9.95
Everything® 30-Minute Sudoku Book, $9.95
**Everything® Bible Crosswords Book, $9.95**
Everything® Blackjack Strategy Book
Everything® Brain Strain Book, $9.95
Everything® Bridge Book
Everything® Card Games Book
Everything® Card Tricks Book, $9.95
Everything® Casino Gambling Book, 2nd Ed.
Everything® Chess Basics Book
Everything® Craps Strategy Book
Everything® Crossword and Puzzle Book
Everything® Crossword Challenge Book
Everything® Crosswords for the Beach Book, $9.95
**Everything® Cryptic Crosswords Book, $9.95**
Everything® Cryptograms Book, $9.95
Everything® Easy Crosswords Book
Everything® Easy Kakuro Book, $9.95
Everything® Easy Large-Print Crosswords Book
Everything® Games Book, 2nd Ed.
Everything® Giant Sudoku Book, $9.95
Everything® Kakuro Challenge Book, $9.95
Everything® Large-Print Crossword Challenge Book
Everything® Large-Print Crosswords Book
Everything® Lateral Thinking Puzzles Book, $9.95

Everything® Literary Crosswords Book, $9.95
Everything® Mazes Book
**Everything® Memory Booster Puzzles Book, $9.95**
Everything® Movie Crosswords Book, $9.95
**Everything® Music Crosswords Book, $9.95**
Everything® Online Poker Book, $12.95
Everything® Pencil Puzzles Book, $9.95
Everything® Poker Strategy Book
Everything® Pool & Billiards Book
**Everything® Puzzles for Commuters Book, $9.95**
Everything® Sports Crosswords Book, $9.95
Everything® Test Your IQ Book, $9.95
Everything® Texas Hold 'Em Book, $9.95
Everything® Travel Crosswords Book, $9.95
**Everything® TV Crosswords Book, $9.95**
Everything® Word Games Challenge Book
Everything® Word Scramble Book
Everything® Word Search Book

## HEALTH

Everything® Alzheimer's Book
Everything® Diabetes Book
Everything® Health Guide to Adult Bipolar Disorder
**Everything® Health Guide to Arthritis**
Everything® Health Guide to Controlling Anxiety
Everything® Health Guide to Fibromyalgia
**Everything® Health Guide to Menopause**
**Everything® Health Guide to OCD**
**Everything® Health Guide to PMS**
Everything® Health Guide to Postpartum Care
Everything® Health Guide to Thyroid Disease
Everything® Hypnosis Book
Everything® Low Cholesterol Book
Everything® Nutrition Book
Everything® Reflexology Book
Everything® Stress Management Book

## HISTORY

Everything® American Government Book
Everything® American History Book, 2nd Ed.
Everything® Civil War Book
Everything® Freemasons Book
Everything® Irish History & Heritage Book
Everything® Middle East Book
Everything® World War II Book, 2nd Ed.

## HOBBIES

Everything® Candlemaking Book
Everything® Cartooning Book
Everything® Coin Collecting Book
Everything® Drawing Book

Everything® Family Tree Book, 2nd Ed.
Everything® Knitting Book
Everything® Knots Book
Everything® Photography Book
Everything® Quilting Book
Everything® Sewing Book
Everything® Soapmaking Book, 2nd Ed.
Everything® Woodworking Book

## HOME IMPROVEMENT

Everything® Feng Shui Book
Everything® Feng Shui Decluttering Book, $9.95
Everything® Fix-It Book
**Everything® Green Living Book**
Everything® Home Decorating Book
Everything® Home Storage Solutions Book
Everything® Homebuilding Book
**Everything® Organize Your Home Book, 2nd Ed.**

## KIDS' BOOKS

All titles are $7.95

Everything® Kids' Animal Puzzle & Activity Book
Everything® Kids' Baseball Book, 4th Ed.
Everything® Kids' Bible Trivia Book
Everything® Kids' Bugs Book
Everything® Kids' Cars and Trucks Puzzle and Activity Book
Everything® Kids' Christmas Puzzle & Activity Book
Everything® Kids' Cookbook
Everything® Kids' Crazy Puzzles Book
Everything® Kids' Dinosaurs Book
**Everything® Kids' Environment Book**
**Everything® Kids' Fairies Puzzle and Activity Book**
Everything® Kids' First Spanish Puzzle and Activity Book
Everything® Kids' Gross Cookbook
Everything® Kids' Gross Hidden Pictures Book
Everything® Kids' Gross Jokes Book
Everything® Kids' Gross Mazes Book
Everything® Kids' Gross Puzzle & Activity Book
Everything® Kids' Halloween Puzzle & Activity Book
Everything® Kids' Hidden Pictures Book
Everything® Kids' Horses Book
Everything® Kids' Joke Book
Everything® Kids' Knock Knock Book
Everything® Kids' Learning Spanish Book
**Everything® Kids' Magical Science Experiments Book**
Everything® Kids' Math Puzzles Book
Everything® Kids' Mazes Book
Everything® Kids' Money Book
Everything® Kids' Nature Book
Everything® Kids' Pirates Puzzle and Activity Book
Everything® Kids' Presidents Book
Everything® Kids' Princess Puzzle and Activity Book
Everything® Kids' Puzzle Book
**Everything® Kids' Racecars Puzzle and Activity Book**
Everything® Kids' Riddles & Brain Teasers Book
Everything® Kids' Science Experiments Book
Everything® Kids' Sharks Book

Everything® Kids' Soccer Book
**Everything® Kids' Spies Puzzle and Activity Book**
Everything® Kids' States Book
Everything® Kids' Travel Activity Book

## KIDS' STORY BOOKS

Everything® Fairy Tales Book

## LANGUAGE

Everything® Conversational Japanese Book with CD, $19.95
Everything® French Grammar Book
Everything® French Phrase Book, $9.95
Everything® French Verb Book, $9.95
Everything® German Practice Book with CD, $19.95
Everything® Inglés Book
Everything® Intermediate Spanish Book with CD, $19.95
**Everything® Italian Practice Book with CD, $19.95**
Everything® Learning Brazilian Portuguese Book with CD, $19.95
**Everything® Learning French Book with CD, 2nd Ed., $19.95**
Everything® Learning German Book
Everything® Learning Italian Book
Everything® Learning Latin Book
**Everything® Learning Russian Book with CD, $19.95**
Everything® Learning Spanish Book with CD, 2nd Ed., $19.95
Everything® Russian Practice Book with CD, $19.95
Everything® Sign Language Book
Everything® Spanish Grammar Book
Everything® Spanish Phrase Book, $9.95
Everything® Spanish Practice Book with CD, $19.95
Everything® Spanish Verb Book, $9.95
Everything® Speaking Mandarin Chinese Book with CD, $19.95

## MUSIC

Everything® Drums Book with CD, $19.95
Everything® Guitar Book with CD, 2nd Ed., $19.95
Everything® Guitar Chords Book with CD, $19.95
Everything® Home Recording Book
Everything® Music Theory Book with CD, $19.95
Everything® Reading Music Book with CD, $19.95
Everything® Rock & Blues Guitar Book with CD, $19.95
Everything® Rock and Blues Piano Book with CD, $19.95
Everything® Songwriting Book

## NEW AGE

Everything® Astrology Book, 2nd Ed.
Everything® Birthday Personology Book
Everything® Dreams Book, 2nd Ed.
Everything® Love Signs Book, $9.95
**Everything® Love Spells Book, $9.95**
Everything® Numerology Book
Everything® Paganism Book
Everything® Palmistry Book
Everything® Psychic Book
Everything® Reiki Book
Everything® Sex Signs Book, $9.95

Everything® Spells & Charms Book, 2nd Ed.
Everything® Tarot Book, 2nd Ed.
Everything® Toltec Wisdom Book
Everything® Wicca and Witchcraft Book

## PARENTING

Everything® Baby Names Book, 2nd Ed.
**Everything® Baby Shower Book, 2nd Ed.**
Everything® Baby's First Year Book
Everything® Birthing Book
Everything® Breastfeeding Book
Everything® Father-to-Be Book
Everything® Father's First Year Book
**Everything® Get Ready for Baby Book, 2nd Ed.**
Everything® Get Your Baby to Sleep Book, $9.95
Everything® Getting Pregnant Book
**Everything® Guide to Pregnancy Over 35**
Everything® Guide to Raising a One-Year-Old
Everything® Guide to Raising a Two-Year-Old
**Everything® Guide to Raising Adolescent Boys**
**Everything® Guide to Raising Adolescent Girls**
Everything® Homeschooling Book
Everything® Mother's First Year Book
Everything® Parent's Guide to Childhood Illnesses
Everything® Parent's Guide to Children and Divorce
Everything® Parent's Guide to Children with ADD/ADHD
Everything® Parent's Guide to Children with Asperger's Syndrome
Everything® Parent's Guide to Children with Autism
Everything® Parent's Guide to Children with Bipolar Disorder
Everything® Parent's Guide to Children with Depression
Everything® Parent's Guide to Children with Dyslexia
Everything® Parent's Guide to Children with Juvenile Diabetes
Everything® Parent's Guide to Positive Discipline
Everything® Parent's Guide to Raising a Successful Child
Everything® Parent's Guide to Raising Boys
Everything® Parent's Guide to Raising Girls
Everything® Parent's Guide to Raising Siblings
Everything® Parent's Guide to Sensory Integration Disorder
Everything® Parent's Guide to Tantrums
Everything® Parent's Guide to the Strong-Willed Child
Everything® Parenting a Teenager Book
Everything® Potty Training Book, $9.95
Everything® Pregnancy Book, 3rd Ed.
Everything® Pregnancy Fitness Book
Everything® Pregnancy Nutrition Book
Everything® Pregnancy Organizer, 2nd Ed., $16.95
Everything® Toddler Activities Book
Everything® Toddler Book
Everything® Tween Book
Everything® Twins, Triplets, and More Book

## PETS

Everything® Aquarium Book
Everything® Boxer Book
Everything® Cat Book, 2nd Ed.
Everything® Chihuahua Book

**Everything® Cooking for Dogs Book**
Everything® Dachshund Book
Everything® Dog Book
Everything® Dog Health Book
Everything® Dog Obedience Book
Everything® Dog Owner's Organizer, $16.95
Everything® Dog Training and Tricks Book
Everything® German Shepherd Book
Everything® Golden Retriever Book
Everything® Horse Book
Everything® Horse Care Book
Everything® Horseback Riding Book
Everything® Labrador Retriever Book
Everything® Poodle Book
Everything® Pug Book
Everything® Puppy Book
Everything® Rottweiler Book
Everything® Small Dogs Book
Everything® Tropical Fish Book
Everything® Yorkshire Terrier Book

## REFERENCE

Everything® American Presidents Book
Everything® Blogging Book
Everything® Build Your Vocabulary Book
Everything® Car Care Book
Everything® Classical Mythology Book
Everything® Da Vinci Book
Everything® Divorce Book
Everything® Einstein Book
Everything® Enneagram Book
Everything® Etiquette Book, 2nd Ed.
**Everything® Guide to Edgar Allan Poe**
Everything® Inventions and Patents Book
Everything® Mafia Book
**Everything® Martin Luther King Jr. Book**
Everything® Philosophy Book
Everything® Pirates Book
Everything® Psychology Book

## RELIGION

Everything® Angels Book
Everything® Bible Book
**Everything® Bible Study Book with CD, $19.95**
Everything® Buddhism Book
Everything® Catholicism Book
Everything® Christianity Book
Everything® Gnostic Gospels Book
Everything® History of the Bible Book
Everything® Jesus Book
Everything® Jewish History & Heritage Book
Everything® Judaism Book
Everything® Kabbalah Book
Everything® Koran Book

Everything® Mary Book
Everything® Mary Magdalene Book
Everything® Prayer Book
Everything® Saints Book, 2nd Ed.
Everything® Torah Book
Everything® Understanding Islam Book
**Everything® Women of the Bible Book**
Everything® World's Religions Book
Everything® Zen Book

## SCHOOL & CAREERS

Everything® Alternative Careers Book
Everything® Career Tests Book
Everything® College Major Test Book
Everything® College Survival Book, 2nd Ed.
Everything® Cover Letter Book, 2nd Ed.
Everything® Filmmaking Book
Everything® Get-a-Job Book, 2nd Ed.
Everything® Guide to Being a Paralegal
Everything® Guide to Being a Personal Trainer
Everything® Guide to Being a Real Estate Agent
Everything® Guide to Being a Sales Rep
**Everything® Guide to Being an Event Planner**
Everything® Guide to Careers in Health Care
Everything® Guide to Careers in Law Enforcement
Everything® Guide to Government Jobs
**Everything® Guide to Starting and Running a Catering Business**
Everything® Guide to Starting and Running a Restaurant
Everything® Job Interview Book
Everything® New Nurse Book
Everything® New Teacher Book
Everything® Paying for College Book
Everything® Practice Interview Book
Everything® Resume Book, 2nd Ed.
Everything® Study Book

## SELF-HELP

**Everything® Body Language Book**
Everything® Dating Book, 2nd Ed.
Everything® Great Sex Book
Everything® Self-Esteem Book
Everything® Tantric Sex Book

## SPORTS & FITNESS

Everything® Easy Fitness Book
**Everything® Krav Maga for Fitness Book**
Everything® Running Book

## TRAVEL

**Everything® Family Guide to Coastal Florida**
Everything® Family Guide to Cruise Vacations
Everything® Family Guide to Hawaii
Everything® Family Guide to Las Vegas, 2nd Ed.
Everything® Family Guide to Mexico
Everything® Family Guide to New York City, 2nd Ed.
Everything® Family Guide to RV Travel & Campgrounds
Everything® Family Guide to the Caribbean
**Everything® Family Guide to the Disneyland® Resort, California Adventure®, Universal Studios®, and the Anaheim Area, 2nd Ed.**
**Everything® Family Guide to the Walt Disney World Resort®, Universal Studios®, and Greater Orlando, 5th Ed.**
Everything® Family Guide to Timeshares
Everything® Family Guide to Washington D.C., 2nd Ed.

## WEDDINGS

Everything® Bachelorette Party Book, $9.95
Everything® Bridesmaid Book, $9.95
Everything® Destination Wedding Book
Everything® Elopement Book, $9.95
Everything® Father of the Bride Book, $9.95
Everything® Groom Book, $9.95
Everything® Mother of the Bride Book, $9.95
Everything® Outdoor Wedding Book
Everything® Wedding Book, 3rd Ed.
Everything® Wedding Checklist, $9.95
Everything® Wedding Etiquette Book, $9.95
Everything® Wedding Organizer, 2nd Ed., $16.95
Everything® Wedding Shower Book, $9.95
Everything® Wedding Vows Book, $9.95
Everything® Wedding Workout Book
**Everything® Weddings on a Budget Book, 2nd Ed., $9.95**

## WRITING

Everything® Creative Writing Book
Everything® Get Published Book, 2nd Ed.
Everything® Grammar and Style Book
Everything® Guide to Magazine Writing
Everything® Guide to Writing a Book Proposal
Everything® Guide to Writing a Novel
Everything® Guide to Writing Children's Books
Everything® Guide to Writing Copy
**Everything® Guide to Writing Graphic Novels**
Everything® Guide to Writing Research Papers
Everything® Screenwriting Book
Everything® Writing Poetry Book
Everything® Writing Well Book